MANAGING RISK DUI COVID-19 PANDE

Global Policies, Narratives and Practices

Andy Alaszewski

With a foreword by
Jens Zinn

First published in Great Britain in 2024 by

Policy Press, an imprint of
Bristol University Press
University of Bristol
1-9 Old Park Hill
Bristol
BS2 8BB
UK
t: +44 (0)117 374 6645
e: bup-info@bristol.ac.uk

Details of international sales and distribution partners are available at
policy.bristoluniversitypress.co.uk

British Library Cataloguing in Publication Data
A catalogue record for this book is available from the British Library

ISBN 978-1-4473-6524-2 hardcover
ISBN 978-1-4473-6525-9 paperback
ISBN 978-1-4473-6526-6 ePub
ISBN 978-1-4473-6527-3 ePdf

Cover design: Nicky Borowiec
Front cover image: Adobe Stock/Zoa-Arts

Bristol University Press and Policy Press use environmentally responsible
print partners.

Printed in Great Britain by CPI Group (UK) Ltd, Croydon, CR0 4YY

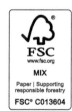

FSC
www.fsc.org
MIX
Paper | Supporting
responsible forestry
FSC® C013604

To my wife, Helen, for being so patient and understanding when I disappear into my head to think or into my room to write.

Contents

List of tables   vi
List of abbreviations   vii
About the author   ix
Acknowledgements   x
Foreword *Jens Zinn*   xi
Preface   xvii

1   Introduction: risk as a key feature of late modern societies   1

PART I   Responding to the challenges of the pandemic
2   Managing uncertainty: framing COVID-19   11
3   The risks of COVID-19: probability, categorisation and outcomes   28
4   Communicating risk: public health messaging   47

PART II   Mitigating risk through science and technology
5   'Following the science': expertise and risk   67
6   Risk work to maintain services during the pandemic   86

PART III Risk narratives
7   Pandemic narratives: telling stories about COVID-19 and its risks   103
8   Contesting risk: conspiracy theories   117
9   Hindsight: inquiries and the blame game   135

10   Conclusion: risk and the pandemic   151

References   162
Index   198

List of tables

2.1	Factors undermining zero-COVID policies	20
3.1	Official categorisation of risk groups and lockdown advice in May 2020	31
3.2	COVID-19 Decision Support Tool	35
3.3	Implications of the precautionary principle	41
4.1	Factors that contribute to the successful communication of risk messages	48
4.2	New Zealand alert system	56
5.1	The network of advisory committees providing expert advice to policy makers in the UK	73
5.2	Relative standing of supporters of aerosol and droplet theories	83
9.1	Timeline for COVID-19-related events in Paznaun valley and Ischgl (February and March 2020)	144

List of abbreviations

ACIP	Advisory Committee on Immunization Practices
BAME	Black and minority ethnic
BCNU	British Columbian Nursing Union
BMA	British Medical Association
BRI	Bristol Royal Infirmary
BSE	Bovine Spongiform Encephalopathy
CDC	Centers for Disease Control and Prevention
CEPI	Coalition of Epidemic Preparedness Innovations
CJD	Creutzfeldt-Jakob Disease
CMO	Chief Medical Officer
COBRA/COBR	Civil Contingencies Committee
COVID-19	Coronavirus Disease 2019
CSA	Chief Scientific Adviser
IC	Intelligence Community of the US
ICU	intensive care unit
ISC	International Science Council
JCVI	Joint Committee on Vaccination and Immunisation
MERS	Middle East Respiratory Syndrome
NERVTAG	New and Emerging Respiratory Virus Threats Advisory Group
NHS	National Health Service
NIAV	National Institute of Allergy and Virology
NICE	National Institute for Health Care and Excellence
NIH	National Institutes for Health
NIHR	National Institute for Health and Care Research
NPHIL	National Public Health Institute Liberia
OECD	Organisation for Economic Co-operation and Development
ONS	Office for National Statistics (UK)
PHE	Public Health England
PPE	personal protective equipment
RCT	randomised control trial
R&D	research and development
SAGE	Scientific Advisory Group for Emergencies
SARS	Severe Acute Respiratory Syndrome
SARS-CoV-2	Severe Acute Respiratory Syndrome Coronavirus 2
SPI	Scientific Advisory Group on Pandemic Influenza
SPI-B	Independent Scientific Pandemic Insights Group on Behaviours

SPI-M	Scientific Pandemic Influenza Group on Modelling
UK	United Kingdom of Great Britain and Northern Ireland
US	United States of America
WHA	World Health Assembly
WHO	World Health Organization

About the author

Andy Alaszewski is Emeritus Professor of Health Studies at the University of Kent. He completed his undergraduate (BA, Social Anthropology) and postgraduate (PhD, Social and Political Sciences) studies at the University of Cambridge. He is an applied social scientist who has researched the ways in which policy decisions are made and implemented, and the role and nature of risk in health and social care. He is the founding Editor of *Health, Risk & Society*, an international peer-reviewed journal published by Taylor & Francis. He is author of numerous scholarly articles, book chapters and books, and is co-author of *Risk, Safety and Clinical Practice: Healthcare through the Lens of Risk* (Heyman et al, 2010) and *Making Health Policy: A Critical Introduction* (Alaszewski and Brown, 2012).

Acknowledgements

I would like to thank my daughter, Anna, for stimulating my interest in how policy makers were responding to COVID-19; my wife, Helen, for reading and critically commenting on the first draft of both this and my earlier book on the subject; and my son, Mark, for his comments. My thanks to MA Healthcare Limited for permission to use material from my article 'Should pregnant women be in a high-risk COVID category' published in the *British Journal of Midwifery* (Alaszewski, 2020a). My thanks to Trish Greenhalgh for allowing me to draw on her study (Greenhalgh, Ozbilgin and Contandriopoulos, 2021) of the scientific dispute over the transmission of SARS-CoV-2 and to use it as a basis for Case Study 6 on the scientific debate about droplet versus aerosol spray modes of transmission.

Foreword

Jens Zinn

Large-scale risks have challenged countries of the global world recently, even more than Ulrich Beck might have imagined when writing about the Risk Society in the mid-1980s. The ongoing debate about climate change has intensified, driven by repeating heatwaves, bushfires and floodings of new intensity, length and frequency. The coronavirus crisis has broken down cognitive divisions between the Global South and the Global North, bringing the awareness that new infectious diseases are a global phenomenon in a world of high mobility. Even before the COVID-19 pandemic has faded, Russia's invasion of parts of Ukraine has resulted in a war that challenges long-term security paradigms, while there is still uncertainty about the Chinese desire to incorporate the technological powerhouse of Taiwan. It is not enough that such large-scale risks challenge societies worldwide. What has been called post-truth (McIntyre, 2018) is characterising a public sphere in turmoil, with traditional information sources losing influence and giving space to both bottom-up social media campaigning and mass manipulation through fake news and conspiracy theories, while the public sphere seems fragmented into echo chambers and epistemic bubbles (Nguyen, 2020). As a result, fundamental social institutions are under pressure, and have to prove their capacity to manage large scale crisis such as the COVID-19 pandemic.

The rise of calculative technologies and their embeddedness in new institutions such as insurance, risk assessment and management, and epidemiology characterises a society that believes in the rational manageability of the future. But, with ongoing modernisation, the side-effects have brought about increasingly more situations where new risks are resistant to technical and economic calculations because they come with multidimensional and systemic uncertainties. These include complexity, lacking knowledge and contradictory interests and values. Consequently, risk is a double-edged sword or an ambivalent concept that stands for the manageability of harm as well as the uncertain catastrophes that inform the current crises we struggle to manage, since innovation rather than past knowledge is the source for its successful management.

The ability of societies to discover risks, the activities that cause side-effects, which are now coming back to haunt us, and their material reality challenge the ways these kinds of crises have been managed in the past. As Alaszewski argues, this is not merely a question of evidence and rational balancing of the options. It is also about socially legitimate ways of dealing with possible harm and responsibility for unpreventable but knowable uncertainties, and cannot be separated from the emotions or intuition and trust, as well as the hope, faith and ideology that accompany the experience of the present and shape the imaginaries of the future (Zinn, 2008, 2016).

A number of sociological approaches have tried to make sense out of the shift towards risk in late modern societies. Most prominently, in the 1980s, Ulrich Beck emphasised the limits of the modern strategies to manage risks giving way and being challenged by the side-effects of successful modernisation processes which now challenges its own institutions (Beck, 1986, 1992). At that time, Mary Douglas developed a cultural approach to understand the different ways in which risks have been, are and will be understood and managed by social entities in the past, present and future at different places throughout the world. Most famous is her cultural theory of risk, which suggests that with the social institutions we cherish we also select the risks we are concerned about (Douglas, 1985, 1990). Scholars developing Foucault's conceptual work on governmentality and biopolitics emphasise how new technologies of power create new ways of governing populations, shaping practices and subjectivities in modern societies (Dean, 1999; Rose, 1990, 2001).

The coronavirus crisis has contributed to changing the debate about mega risks. Early sociological work on risk were driven by the civil use of nuclear power and early accidents such as at Three Mile Island, which stimulated research on risk and complex technologies. HIV/AIDS shifted the focus to individual and collective responses to this new illness, bringing into focus the discrimination of homosexuals within most Western societies. 9/11 has fostered security studies and the possibilities that voluntarily produced risks will harm others, as with the current war in the Ukraine. The COVID-19 pandemic brought into light the broad global dimension that shapes the development of the risk, and also highlighted how national responses in the global world increase social divisions and interrupt global networks of work, production and care. It therefore showed the need for, and pressed for, global collaboration and a cosmopolitan approach, but at the same time showed how colonialism, global inequalities and national prejudice can still hinder an efficient approach to pandemics.

Alaszewski's book shows, with the example of the unfolding coronavirus crisis, the value of going beyond the orthodoxy of mainstream macro-theories on risk to look at the concrete empirical reality of a specific case. *Managing Risk during the COVID-19 Pandemic: Global Policies, Narratives and Practices* provides an original contribution to the debate as well as a personal account of the author's own experience and involvement in epidemics, advising as a public health expert. As did many others, he wondered 'why most governments in Europe were slow to react, given that the warning signs were there from mid-January'. This has resulted in a book that combines social science risk studies with a public health perspective, giving an account of the unfolding of the crisis specifically in the UK but systematically embedding this narrative in the unfolding and management of the crisis elsewhere in the world. Rather than being overly sociological, getting buried in theoretical considerations or getting lost in the mass of data and experiences, Alaszewski provides a pragmatic selection of key issues, underpinning present-day and historical data and illustrative case studies to develop his argument.

Alaszewski observes that countries can be distinguished according to two fundamentally different ways of understanding the illness, either as a SARS- or Ebola-like virus, emphasising its lethal aspects and adopting zero-COVID-policies, or as a flu-like virus, and therefore engaging in wait-and-see policies while warning individuals to protect themselves.

Introducing the concept of framing, the author suggests that these different ways of viewing the pandemic go back to earlier experiences in countries with SARS and Ebola in Asia, the Middle East and Africa and the flu in Europe and North America; these experiences resulted in very different understandings and responses right from the beginning. These frames were also supported by institutions and their practices, which had been established during earlier disease management and were therefore relatively stable, but he also shows by examples the conditions under which they could be challenged, as in the US. However, frames only capture key elements of an issue and never the whole reality. Both the flu frame and the SARS frame worked well for parts of COVID-19, but the virus's behaviour also deviated. It spread twice as fast as SARS, and much of this was hidden by presymptomatic and asymptomatic transmission. While flu-based approaches underestimated the spread of the virus, zero-COVID countries, which had been successful at the beginning, had later difficulties in finding an exit strategy while other countries still had high infection rates and new virus variants.

Alaszewski also argues that pandemic responses should be underpinned by different values. Triage systems, for example, come with a bias towards younger and healthy populations, which has raised concerns that groups of people with health issues could be disadvantaged. As a whole, the wait-and-see approach as applied by the UK government prioritises normal life for younger people over protecting older and other vulnerable groups. Similar patterns are identified by Alaszewski in the vaccination strategies. Governments that focused on vaccinating younger and economically active people were willing to tolerate serious illness and death among vulnerable groups. Prioritising high risk groups accepted the continued disruption of the lives of younger people to protect the lives of those who were more vulnerable if infected. That people in everyday life balance multiple risks and opportunities is key to understanding what is missing in public health experts' approach to pandemics, with their focus on the dangers of specific illnesses. Lockdown-measures, for example, may reduce some risks while significantly increasing others, as Alaszewski shows with the example of pregnancy, arguing that 'policy makers (inadvertently) contributed to their increased anxiety and depression, and reduced their capacity to manage the different risks they [pregnant women] faced'.

Acknowledging that deaths during a pandemic are inevitable is necessary in order to set political priorities. However, many politicians were unwilling to express this openly, and therefore tended to shift such decisions to experts – suggesting that they were 'following the science'. However, they used the evidence only as long as it did not interfere with their values. Experts, for example in the UK and US, therefore became frustrated as their advice was ignored.

The book turns to the key issue of how to communicate to the public during a crisis, suggesting the need to find a balance between creating enough and too little anxiety so that people comply with recommended individual responses. Trust is a well-known central element for successful risk communication, as many studies have argued for decades. Trust is as much a result of and not just a prerequisite for good risk management, as the examples of New Zealand and Hong Kong show (Chan, 2021).

But why did some evidence find it easier to break through? Alaszewski argues, using the example of recommendations to wear a face mask, that expert groups' access to politicians varied. Proponents of the mainstream droplet theory who were sceptical of face masks as a means of tackling the coronavirus were well connected to politics, while experts of different disciplines who suggested that transmission would take place through aerosol had to use open letters, articles in journals and newspapers, and postings on social media and tweets before their views were recognized.

The reality of the virus required politicians to respond. Its ability to spread quickly endangered the health system, which could be overwhelmed not only by a large number of patients but also by infected staff. This upturned the relationship between the health-care system and the rest of society. The health-care systems themselves and their staff had to be protected by locking down social and economic activity.

Public awareness of the COVID-19 pandemic was to a large degree mediated through risk narratives produced by different social players and the media. Commentators using historically developed risk matrices, which provided evidence about the unfolding of the crisis, tried to make sense of the pandemic by presenting data and explaining it. At the same time, the media added moral judgements and emotion to the numbers and facts by showing what they meant for people's everyday lives. Personal stories are a key medium through which the media communicate risk (Kitzinger, 1999). Journalists used official sources and statistics to identify disadvantaged groups that experienced disproportionate levels of infections and deaths, and added personal stories 'to illustrate the emotions, such as sadness and loss, and moral implications, especially the injustice of such illnesses and deaths'. From a phenomenological perspective, such personal accounts of pandemic risks provide a sense of immediately felt truth in contrast to the abstract accounts of experts and politicians who are managing populations (Schulz and Zinn, 2022).

However, inconsistent risk communication by politicians supports mistrust in traditional media. Many people turned to social media, where it was easy to access fake news and conspiracy theories. These connected to established discourses on 'the poor people' versus the 'corrupt elite', supporting suspicion about government crisis responses. Such suspicions were amplified by politicians' non-compliance with regulations, such as Dominic Cummings's non-compliance with lockdown regulations in the UK in March 2020.

The management of responsibility or the blame game is a key element of any public risk management. Politicians are well aware of the dangers of responsibilisation, and try to evade being made responsible for undesirable outcomes. Therefore, public inquiries serve as much to deflect blame and justify actions by external authorities as they do to scrutinise the management of a crisis.

Alaszewski concludes that "Risk assessment is a way of making predictions about the future, and thus it can form the basis of rational decision making – but only if decision makers are able to access and are willing to use this knowledge.' The crucial question therefore remains how. under crisis conditions, governments can put institutional, cultural and economic preconditions aside to prioritise efficient risk management, and how risk communication in the public sphere can be supported by politicians and the media alike. Looking at democratic societies, controversial debate seems to be part of the negotiation of risk and values that guides responses. It may thus be the acknowledgement and navigation of uncertainty rather than the quick reduction and invisibilisation of it that allows us to be open to new knowledge, differing experiences and innovative responses.

References

Beck, U. (1986) *Risikogesellschaft: auf dem Weg in eine andere Moderne* (1. Aufl. ed.), Frankfurt am Main: Suhrkamp.

Beck, U. (1992) *Risk Society: Towards a New Modernity*, London, Newbury Park, CA: Sage Publications.

Chan, R.K. (2021) 'Tackling COVID-19 risk in Hong Kong: examining distrust, compliance and risk management', *Current Sociology*, 69(4): 547–565. doi:10.1177/0011392121990026

Dean, M. (1999) *Governmentality: Power and Rule in Modern Society*, London: Sage.

Douglas, M. (1985) *Risk Acceptability according to the Social Sciences* (Vol. 11), New York: Russell Sage Foundation.

Douglas, M. (1990) 'Risk as a forensic resource', *DAEDALUS*, 119(4): 1–16.

Kitzinger, J. (1999) 'Researching risk and the media', *Health, Risk & Society*, 1(1): 55–69.

McIntyre, L. (2018) *Post-Truth*, Cambridge, MA: MIT Press.

Nguyen, C.T. (2020) 'Echo chambers and epistemic bubbles', *Episteme*, 17(2): 141–161. doi:10.1017/epi.2018.32

Rose, N. (1990) *Governing the Soul: The Shaping of the Private Self*, London: Routledge.

Rose, N. (2001) 'The politics of life itself', *Theory, Culture & Society*, 18(6): 1–30.

Schulz, M. and Zinn, J.O. (2022). 'Rationales of risk and uncertainty and their epistemological foundation by new phenomenology', *Journal of Risk Research*, https://doi.org/10.1080/13669877.2022.2162105

Zinn, J.O. (2008) 'Heading into the unknown: everyday strategies for managing risk and uncertainty', *Health, Risk & Society*, 10(5), 439–450. doi:10.1080/13698570802380891

Zinn, J.O. (2016) '"In-between" and other reasonable ways to deal with risk and uncertainty: a review article', *Health, Risk & Society*, 18(7–8): 348–366. doi:10.1080/13698575.2016.1269879

Preface

This book developed out of my interest in risk. Since the mid-1990s, I have concentrated my academic work on risk and society.

In 2008, I was invited to join the UK Scientific Advisory Group on Pandemic Influenza (SPI) convened by the Department of Health, a precursor of the current scientific advisory groups on pandemics. At committee meetings, we considered the risk and impact of a global flu pandemic on the UK (high) and the effectiveness of possible responses (probably limited). The three groups of experts on the committee each advocated a different approach to reducing the risk of a pandemic:

- Scientists with expertise in microbiology or pharmacy supported the development of vaccines to prevent infection or mitigate symptoms. This can be problematic as flu and other viruses tend to mutate rapidly, so vaccines have limited efficacy against new variants.
- Behavioural scientists advocated behavioural changes, such as improving personal hygiene, covering coughs and sneezes, and hand washing. It was not clear how easy it would be to improve personal hygiene or how effective these measures would be in limiting the spread of a highly infectious virus that spread from person to person by aerosol spray.
- Epidemiologists and risk experts (I formed part of this group) focused more on evidence from past pandemics, especially the 1918–1919 Spanish flu pandemic and the role that reducing social contact played in reducing the spread of the virus. In the US, cities that shut down and reduced social activity quickly and stayed shut down the longest had the lowest death rates, whereas cities that did not shut down or delayed shutting down and reopened quite quickly had a higher death rate.

During a pandemic, the global spread of a deadly disease, it was probable that the virus causing the disease would be carried into the UK by international travellers and then distributed by public transport systems and large-scale gatherings. The most effective way of controlling its spread was to control access through ports and airports and to reduce social interactions on public transport and at large public events. In a pandemic, it would be important to warn the public, especially the most vulnerable such as older people, so they could take action to protect themselves.

The civil servants who supported the committee were unreceptive to controlling movement and social distancing. They felt that such collective action would infringe on civil liberties and disrupt economic activity. They were more receptive to approaches that focused on individuals: vaccination and personal hygiene measures.

Becoming aware of COVID-19

I first became aware of COVID-19 in early 2020. My wife Helen's brother was admitted to a major teaching hospital in Paris in early February 2020 with advanced kidney cancer, and died in April 2020. Through February into early March, we visited him regularly and observed the French response to COVID-19, including social distancing and mask wearing. When we returned to England in early March, I was shocked at the lack of action. Despite media reports that there were virus hotspots in Northern Italy and central Spain, and that the virus was rapidly spreading in Europe, the UK government was not monitoring travellers from these hotspots or restricting public gatherings. In early March, it seemed to be encouraging such gatherings: on 7 March Boris Johnson, the UK prime minister, and his fiancée Carrie Symonds were part of a crowd of over 67,000 spectators watching the England versus Scotland rugby match at Twickenham.

Writing an e-book

I found it difficult to see why most governments in Europe were slow to react, given that the warning signs were there from mid-January. This stimulated my interest in the pandemic, and is one reason why I decided to write this book.

Another stimulus came a couple of weeks later. On 16 March, I was listening to the 6 o'clock news on BBC Radio 4 when I heard the Chief Medical Officer (CMO), Chris Whitty, identify a number of groups who were at high risk and should protect themselves, including pregnant women. My daughter, Anna, who was pregnant and lived in New York, had heard the same interview, and phoned me to talk about it. To be sure that I understood what Chris Whitty had said, I watched the briefing on YouTube. I was able to reassure Anna that it was a precautionary measure and there was no evidence that she or her unborn baby were especially vulnerable to COVID-19. However, I was curious as to why the precautionary principle of 'better safe than sorry' was being used to include pregnant women in the high-risk category.

In March 2021, Policy Press published an e-book (Alaszewski, 2021a) based on my analysis of the ways in which different countries framed and managed risk in the first year of the pandemic. At the time, the second wave of the virus was at its peak in the UK and was still spreading globally. Even countries that had successfully adopted a zero COVID-19 policy, such as Taiwan, South Korea, Australia and New Zealand, were experiencing localised outbreaks. However the successful development and roll-out of COVID-19 vaccines seemed to offer a way out of the pandemic.

Updating the book to take into account vaccination and other developments

In July 2021, Policy Press offered me the opportunity to update and develop the e-book. I was delighted to accept this opportunity as it enabled me to reflect on the changes in the later stages of the pandemic, especially in terms of the following:

- The emergence of variants: SAR-CoV-2 is a small sequence of genetic material that accumulates errors, some enabling it to infect more efficiently or cause more or less serious illness. Over time, these mutations replace other types and become the dominant variants. The new variants developed in areas with high infection rates such as the UK (Alpha, September 2020), South Africa (Beta, October 2020), Brazil (Gamma, late 2020), India (Delta, late 2020) and South Africa (Omicron, November 2021) (WHO, 2021a).
- The impact of COVID-19 vaccines: Several vaccines were approved for use by the end of 2020, and by the end of 2021, early adopting countries had fully vaccinated those adults willing to be vaccinated and started to vaccinate children. As the levels of vaccination increased, so their impact became evident. In most countries, vaccination substantially reduced the severity of infection, reducing hospitalisations and deaths, but had less impact on transmission.
- The global dimension: COVID-19 became a global pandemic, but for the most part the responses were national. Countries pursued their own self-interest with little regard to the impact this might have on other countries or on the overall development of the pandemic.
- Repeating the same errors: It is relatively easy to understand why policy makers in some countries were slow to react and made errors in their initial assessment of the risk of COVID-19. However, it is more difficult to explain why these policy makers continued to make the same mistakes, responding too slowly to the danger of rising infection and being too eager to remove protections when infection rates started falling.

Andy Alaszewski
Canterbury, Kent
November 2022

Introduction: risk as a key feature of late modern societies

Managing uncertainty: dangers and misfortunes

All societies need to manage the uncertainties of the future and account for the misfortunes of the past. In pre-modern societies, religious and supernatural beliefs, whether in sin, magic or witchcraft (Alaszewski, 2015), provided the basis for prediction of the future and allocation of blame for misfortunes. In modern high-income countries with developed health-care systems, such beliefs have been (partially) replaced by the use of rationality, especially risk, making it possible for human actions to be based on reason and evidence. Indeed, for sociologists such as Anthony Giddens (1990, p. 20), rationality is one of the defining characteristics of modernity.

Measuring risk to manage uncertainty

The emergence of risk evaluation as a framework for rational decision making can be traced back to 17th-century commercial and leisure activities. Merchants developed the mechanism of insurance for managing the uncertainties of shipping, with Lloyd's of London being founded by Edward Lloyd in a coffee shop in London in 1686: it still functions as a marketplace in which insurers pool and share risk. Leisure activities such as gambling provided the mathematical underpinning of risk assessment, with statistics and probability developing out of studies of games of chance (Bernstein, 1996). In the 18th century, the study and use of risk was stimulated by the Enlightenment, a social movement committed to the development of secular knowledge that aimed to replace ignorance, superstition and religion with rationality based on science. Risk provided a way of rationally linking the past, present and future: by observing past events, it was possible to calculate the probability of such events occurring in the future, and therefore make better, more rational decisions in the present (Bernstein, 1996, p. 48).

Predicting the future

A key role of risk assessment is to provide a way of reducing uncertainty by predicting the future, especially identifying dangers that can be avoided. This is often seen as a technical exercise based on measuring the probability of outcomes. During the COVID-19 pandemic, a lot of attention was given to measuring or modelling the probability of infection by the virus.

Less attention tends to be paid to the other key elements of risk assessment, which are measuring and valuing outcomes. When focusing on one specific outcome, such as contracting COVID-19, the values are clear: contracting COVID-19 is a bad outcome, and it is self-evident that reducing infection and 'saving lives' is a positive outcome. However, things become complex when choices have to be made that involve a good outcome for some individuals but a bad outcome for others. In September 2020, Dominic Cummings, a former policy adviser, accused the UK prime minister of delaying lockdown in September 2020 because most of those dying were over 80: while a lockdown would protect older vulnerable people, it would harm younger people (BBC, 2021a). The Prime Minister's Office issued an immediate and widely reported rebuttal of this value judgement, asserting that the prime minister had made rational decisions and that he had taken the 'necessary action to protect lives and livelihoods, guided by the best scientific advice' (BBC, 2021a, np).

As I will argue in Chapters 3 and 5, policy makers are more comfortable dealing with the technical aspects of risk, the numbers, but are less comfortable when choices have to be made between different outcomes, as these involve making value judgements.

Trust and hope

Risk evaluation and rational decision making are aspirations. Individuals in modern societies, especially those in positions of power who make decisions on behalf of others, seek to legitimise their authority by claiming that their decisions are rational, based on the best possible evidence and on risk assessments, and will result in the best possible outcomes (Alaszewski and Brown, 2012). However, there are a number of factors that undermine rationality. Perhaps the most obvious of these is a lack of knowledge. As I show in Chapter 2, at the start of the pandemic, policy makers had to deal with the uncertainty of a new disease. In the absence of evidence from the past, they had to find new ways of thinking about and making sense of the future. One way of doing this is to frame the new situation as similar to one in the past. As I argue in Chapter 2 the way in which COVID-19 was framed had important consequences.

In modern societies, knowledge about complex events such as pandemics tends to be controlled by technical experts, scientists and professionals. Most policy makers and most citizens are not experts, and therefore depend on and have to trust experts (Alaszewski, 2003). Trust involves an element of rationality. Individuals can use different sources of information to judge trustworthiness, such as their past experience, the recommendation of friends and family, evidence of qualifications or personal judgement. But trust also has a non-rational element: it is essentially an act or leap of faith in which the unknowable is disregarded or discounted (Möllering, 2001, p. 403). Trust is a way of managing uncertainty and avoiding the paralysing complexity of rationally analysing every possible future. As Brown and Calnan (2012) observe, individuals who have to deal with challenging situations often have a will to trust. As I demonstrate in Chapter 4, effective communication between policy makers and the public depends on trust and during the pandemic the actions of policy makers in some countries undermined this trust. Such distrust is problematic as policy makers have access to risk assessments and want to communicate them to the members of the public so they can change their behaviours in ways that reduces individual and collective risk. In Chapter 3, I examine how policy makers communicated the risks of COVID-19 and how this influenced trust in different countries.

In most policy systems, politicians who take on responsibility for policy making in health do not have specific expertise in health (in the UK, it is unusual to have a health minister with experience of health and social care). Therefore, these politicians have to rely on scientists and medical specialists who do have this expertise. As I show in Chapter 6, such relationships may be difficult, and indeed there may be an element of mistrust, especially where there is a conflict of ideologies.

Trust and hope are essentially default strategies, used when there is a knowledge deficit. There are other strategies that exist alongside them and can undermine or come into conflict with risk-based strategies, including faith, ideology and emotion (Zinn, 2008).

Limits of rationality and risk

Risk assessment is based on calculations, the systematic use of reason based on evidence. This can be both time-consuming and demanding. In everyday life, such systematic approaches are often bypassed by the use of shortcuts such as emotions, intuition, heuristics and rule of thumb. Unlike arguments based on reason and rationality, emotional appeals do not require a lot of thought or effort to understand; they can easily be converted into and communicated as slogans. Public health campaigners have used emotional appeals to foreground particular health risks, thereby altering individuals' behaviour by making them more aware of and anxious about specific threats to their health. Emotions can also be exploited for other, less benign purposes. When the pandemic began, a number of countries had right-wing populist leaders (US, UK and Brazil), whose divisive politics were based on emotional appeals to their base and scapegoating of opponents, including experts.

Risk evaluation and society

Risk initially developed as a way of predicting the future and providing protection from the inevitable misfortunes of trading. For Enlightenment thinkers, it provided a way of creating a more rational society through science- and evidence-based decisions. However, in the late 20th century, social scientists developed more critical awareness of the ways in which risk is embedded in key social processes and influences social relations and interactions. This more critical approach is evident in Beck and Giddens's analyses of the key features of late modern societies, or so-called Risk Society; it is also an important element in Douglas's cultural theory and forms part of Foucault's analysis of power or governmentality in modern societies.

Beck, Giddens and Risk Society

Beck (1992) argues that in late modern or Risk Society, traditional forms of social structuring based on occupation, social class and wealth have to some extent been replaced by structuring based on exposures to risk, especially manufactured risks – by-products of the technologies used in modern societies. Unlike the risks of pre-modern societies, which were often localised and clearly marked, many of the risks of modernity are invisible, examples being air pollution and radiation, and can only be identified by special technologies. Modern risks are also global. The 1986 meltdown of a nuclear reactor in Chernobyl contaminated grasslands 3,000 miles away in the Lake District, and sheep were still being tested for radiation poisoning 30 years later (*Cumberland News*, 2016).

Beck and Giddens argue that protection from risk in modern society depends more on knowledge than wealth. To protect themselves, individuals need to access the technologies and information through which they can identify and mitigate risks, a process Giddens refers to as reflexivity (1991, p. 2). In Chapter 3, I consider how the government provided information to enable individuals to identify risk and take measures to protect themselves.

As Gabe (2021) observes, Beck's Risk Society hypothesis was grounded in growing public scepticism of the claims that scientific and technological progress created safer and more secure societies. Gabe notes that this scepticism reflected 'the failure of regulatory institutions to manage major risk incidents and fears regarding the effects of rapidly developing science, such as the production of genetically modified foods, human cloning, and nanotechnology' (2021, p. 535). In Chapter 8, I examine COVID-19 conspiracy theories, one of the major signs that government and scientists are mistrusted.

Mary Douglas, blame and the social construction of risk

In his early work, Beck views risk as a social reality, an objective fact that has social implications. Mary Douglas (1990) observes that while dangers and hazards exist in any given setting, some hazards are selected for attention and mitigating action while others are disregarded. Indeed in some contexts, risks are created that do not relate to 'real' hazards. Beck treats risk as a modern phenomenon. Douglas in contrast observes that while risk may be a modern phenomenon, other concepts, such as sin, play a similar role in other cultures (Douglas, 1990). Both sin and risk can be used to control behaviour by establishing the norms of social behaviour and allocating blame and sanctions if these norms are transgressed. Douglas notes that both risk and sin operate in and through time. She argues that before a bad event, the sinner about to sin or risk-taker about to take a risk is warned of the dangers. If these warnings are ignored and the predicted bad event happens, then the sinner or risk-taker is blamed for failing to heed the warnings (Douglas, 1990, p. 5). As Lupton notes, in Douglas's analysis of risk, every accident and misfortune —especially when they result in death – must be 'chargeable to someone's account'; someone must be blamed (Lupton 1999, p. 45).

The disregarding of warnings and subsequent allocation of blame can be seen in various modern disasters. In the case of Bovine Spongiform Encephalopathy/Variant Creutzfeldt–Jakob disease (BSE/vCJD, so-called mad cow disease and its human version), Richard Lacey, a microbiologist, was a dissenting scientist whose warnings that BSE could and would infect humans were ridiculed (BMJ, 2019). In 1996, the government had to admit that BSE had infected humans, and appointed a team to investigate the failure to identify and mitigate this risk. In Annex 2 of their report (BSE Inquiry, 2000, p. 5), the team allocated responsibility to named individuals for their failure to identify that eating infected meat would harm humans. In Chapter 9, I consider the role of blame in the pandemic and the role of public inquiries in examining ways in which policy makers failed to identify and take measures to mitigate the risks of COVID-19.

Douglas sees blaming and ascribing dangerous polluting powers to individuals and groups who threaten ordered society as a universal phenomenon. As she notes (Douglas, 1966), in many social settings there is a struggle to maintain and protect purity from the ever encroaching threat of pollution. When impurity threatens to breach the boundary protecting purity, that boundary has to be reinforced and protected. For example, there are traditional cultural beliefs in Japan that the boundaries of the body need to be protected from pollution, with the throat being the major portal – a crucial border that needs special protection. In the 2009 swine flu epidemic, the Japanese government extended the World Health Organization (WHO) guidelines for prevention of transmission, adding gargling and mask wearing. The Ministry of Health undertook large public health campaigns encouraging the Japanese to *tearai* (hand wash), *ugai* (gargle) and *masku* (wear protective masks) (Armstrong-Hough, 2015, p. 287). In Japan mask wearing has previously been used to protect the body against other dangers. Burgess and Horii (2012) note that following the Fukushima nuclear accident in 2011, mask wearing was used as a protection against radiation. As I show in Chapter 8, there was a very different cultural response in Europe and North America, with considerable resistance to public health messaging encouraging mask wearing.

Michel Foucault, risk and professional discourses

Like Douglas, Foucault sees risk as a social construct. He is interested in the way risk has been used as a means of social control, initially based on analysis of historical studies of the ways in which societies responded to the risk posed by social deviance (Foucault, 1967). He observes that in Europe before the 19th century deviance was visibly and publicly controlled; for example, the punishment of criminals was a public spectacle. Reformers argued that such responses were inhumane and inefficient, and advocated reforms in which social deviants were separated and reformed in institutions. In the early 19th century, major programmes of construction in Europe and North America created asylums to incarcerate those seen as risks: paupers, lunatics and criminals.

Such a major change in defining and responding to risk was well documented, but it was usually characterised as a benign reform that drew on the progressive ideas of the 18th century. The role of Revolutionary France in pioneering many of the reforms gave credence to the idea that they were a product of more enlightened thinking. For example, Phillipe Pinel, reformed the treatment of the mentally ill in Paris by removing the chains that restrained them (Foucault, 1967, p. 469). In these new institutions, professionals exercised social authority and detailed control over inmates' lives. Such power was justified as being in their interest as it would help to reform them.

Foucault argues that the new institutions represented a new form of disciplinary power. They were not just a practical way of managing the increasing number of individuals who were causing a nuisance in the expanding urban centres of the Industrial Revolution, but they were also a source of new knowledge and a new way of defining and understanding danger. The professionals who managed these institutions claimed, and were given, the right to identify the 'abnormal' and separate them. They could study, identify and name different types of abnormality, examine their causes and ways in which they could be treated. This process created a distinctive expert language or discourse. In 1798, Pinel published his classification or nosology of diseases that identified four types of mental disorder: melancholia, mania (with or without delirium), dementia and idiocy. This approach is still evident in the more fine-grained classification of mental disorders in the American Psychiatric Association's *Diagnostic and Statistical Manual of Mental Disorders*, first published in 1952 and regularly updated (Holmes and Warelow, 1999, p. 167).

Starr refers to the power of experts, such as medical professionals, to define a specific type of abnormality or risk as cultural authority; 'the probability that particular definitions of reality and judgments of meaning and value will prevail as valid and true' (Starr, 1982, p. 13).

While institutions such as hospitals provide the cases that doctors can use to identify diseases and their symptoms, the development of epidemiology has enabled doctors to identify the community settings in which particular diseases develop. Armstrong (1995) argues that 'this type of evidence changes the nature of illness, through the novel and pivotal medical concept of *risk*. It is no longer the symptom or sign [in the body] pointing tantalisingly at the hidden pathological truth of disease, but the risk factor opening up a space of future illness potential [in the community]' (emphasis in the original, Armstrong, 1995, p. 400).

Increased knowledge about the factors influencing the development of disease have undermined the binary divide between health and illness, replacing it with a risk/disease continuum, for example in the concept of 'pre-diabetes'. If an individual has a blood test that identifies raised blood sugar level, then their doctor may warn them that they are at risk of developing diabetes, and label them as 'pre-diabetic' – neither healthy nor ill (Hindhede, 2014). Aronowitz (2009) refers to this as a new pre-disease state that effectively medicalises the previously healthy. He observes that there has been a convergence between risk and disease, especially for chronic disease, creating a hybrid situation in which the management of the disease is oriented towards risk, towards the reduction of possible harmful outcomes: 'In many instances, chronic disease has become a kind of risk state in which diagnosis, treatment, and "disease management" are directed at reducing the chances of anticipated, feared developments' (Aronowitz, 2009, p. 419). The grouping together of those at risk with those who have diagnosed symptoms creates a risk/disease population. As I show in Chapter 3, identifying at-risk individuals played an important role in government warnings about the threat of COVID-19 and in lockdown policies, which some countries were forced to adopt and effectively made whole populations into COVID-19 risk/disease populations subject to legal/medical surveillance and control.

Foucault's analysis of the ways in which professional discourses create and maintain the barrier between normality and abnormality and structure the ways in which risk is defined and managed, highlights the key role that experts and their discourses play in structuring risk. In Chapters 5 and 6, I consider the key role that experts, especially doctors, played in the pandemic, both in providing the knowledge that shaped responses and in delivering the front-line services that exposed them to stress and danger.

Comment

In modern society, risk plays a key role in individual and collective decision making. It provides a way of predicting future and accounting for past mistakes. As I will show in this remainder of this book, the sudden global spread of SARS-CoV-2 created serious challenges, which policy makers in different countries met with varying success.

This sudden global crisis offers an opportunity to reflect on the ways in which risk provides insights into the development of contemporary societies. Beck and Giddens's Risk Society theory highlights the ways in individuals are threatened by new and global risks and how they need to draw on expert knowledge to identify and manage those risks. Mary Douglas's cultural theory highlights the ways in which risk is socially constructed, and the ways in which such construction reflects cultural values and beliefs about the sources of danger. Foucault's analysis of the role of professionals and their discourses highlights the key role they play in structuring risk evaluation in contemporary societies, and how these discourses conceal power and control over everyday life and activities in contemporary societies.

PART I

Responding to the challenges of the pandemic

2

Managing uncertainty: framing COVID-19

Responding to the developing challenges of a new infectious disease

Risk and framing

In early 2020, COVID-19 was a new disease, so there was no evidence on which to base an assessment of risk. One way of dealing with this uncertainty was to equate the new disease with an existing disease, a process that can be referred to as framing. Goffman (1975) argues that when faced with a puzzling or novel situation, individuals have to decide 'What is going on here?', and framing enables them to do this. When framing a new phenomenon, individuals and groups draw on their knowledge of similar events or situations. A significant event that attracted substantial public and media attention can become a reference point and a frame for similar events in the future. If the original event is linked to a name or phrase, then this is used when framing subsequent events. For example, since President Nixon's resignation in 1974 following the burglary of the Democratic National Committee headquarters in Watergate Office Building, the suffix 'gate' has referred to alleged illegal events that have been covered up, such as Partygate, the breaches of COVID-19 lockdown rules at the UK prime minister's residence (O'Grady, 2022). Aronowitz (2008) notes that framing a disease is a way of recognising, defining, naming and categorising it, and attributing it to a cause or set of causes. Such framing shapes individual and collective responses (2008, p. 2).

The development and maintenance of frames

Framing is influenced by the interests of individuals and groups. For example, when the aircraft manufacturer Boeing launched a new aircraft, the 737 Max, it was in its interest to frame it as a minor modification of the 737 rather than a new design, as this reduced the costs of regulatory approval. This framing was accepted both by the regulatory authority, minimising scrutiny, and by the airlines, minimising pilot retraining. As a congressional inquiry made clear, the new plane was actually significantly different and had a basic design flaw 'that resulted in the tragic and preventable deaths of 346 people' (The House Committee on Transportation and Infrastructure, 2020, p. 5).

Once a frame has become established, it can be difficult to change, especially when it is accepted by a social group – forming the basis of their decision making and acting as a device to filter out adverse criticism. To take just one example, at Bristol Royal Infirmary there were major shortcomings among paediatric surgeons between 1984 and 1995, resulting in at least 34 excess deaths in paediatric heart surgery (see Spiegelhalter et al, 2002). Despite internal complaints and articles in the media referring to 'dismal mortality statistics in the paediatric cardiac surgery unit since 1988' (BBC, 1999), senior managers and surgeons maintained that the unit was a centre of excellence and that the mortality figures were a product of the complexity of cases they had to manage. They filtered out adverse criticism through a 'club culture' that labelled critics as troublemakers. It took disciplinary action by the General Medical Council and a national inquiry (BRI Inquiry, 2001) to shift the framing of events in the unit, but as Kewell (2006, p. 374) observes, despite this shift to a 'under-performance, risk, and danger' frame, senior managers and surgeons tried to maintain the 'safety and excellence' frame in their evidence.

Framing COVID-19: the policy implications

In early 2020, as information about a new form of pneumonia of unknown origins started to come out of China, policy makers round the world had to answer a question: what sort of disease is COVID-19? They answered this in different ways, and these different answers had important policy implications.

The framing of COVID-19 in early 2020

The way policy makers framed COVID-19 was shaped by their experience of infectious diseases. In the western Pacific Rim and parts of Africa, epidemics of infectious lethal diseases such as SARS and Ebola shaped responses, while in Europe and North America policy makers were more familiar with seasonal flu, which is highly infectious but is usually a mild illness except for vulnerable individuals.

SARS, Ebola and rapid response zero-COVID policies

Since the start of the new millennium, there had been a number of epidemics of infectious and lethal diseases: Severe Acute Respiratory Syndrome (SARS) in 2003, Middle East Respiratory Syndrome (MERS) 2012 and 2015, and Ebola in 2013. These outbreaks were caused by the mutation of a virus, which enabled it to spread in human populations. While outbreaks tended to be localised and contained by public health measures, air travel facilitated the spread of viruses and international outbreaks. For example,

MERS originated and was originally contained in Jordan and the Arabian peninsula, but in 2015 there was an outbreak in South Korea. In countries directly affected by these diseases, policy makers were altered to the dangers and the need to prepare for another similar disease. For example, following the SARS outbreak, Taiwan identified the need for a disaster management centre that could rapidly respond to large outbreaks of infectious disease and coordinate a national response that communicated and coordinated with national, regional and local authorities. In 2004, the Taiwanese government established a National Health Command Center to fulfil this role (Taiwan CDC, 2018). In South Korea, the uncoordinated national response to MERS in 2015 (Kim et al, 2021) stimulated a rethink of national policies and a programme of reform to improve preparedness and response. At national level, the government established an Emergency Operation Center within the Center for Disease Control and Prevention (CDC). The CDC's director was incorporated within national policy making as a vice-minister. Laboratory capacity was expanded to enable large-scale testing for a new disease, five regional centres were established and there was an increase in disease response staff. An active programme of monitoring infectious diseases outside Korea was implemented, with monitoring at ports of entry and facilities for quarantining suspect cases (Yang et al, 2021).

Countries with direct experience of SARS or similar diseases framed COVID-19 as similar to SARS; as a highly infectious and lethal disease that could be eliminated by public health measures. They focused on controlling the virus and preventing its spread through zero-COVID policies. They were proactive, trying to prevent the virus entering their country by monitoring travellers from viral hotspots, and breaking the chain of transmission by rapidly identifying and isolating infected individuals and their contacts if the virus eluded these measures (Llupià et al, 2020).

Zero-COVID policies were adopted by countries in the western Pacific Rim. In Taiwan, where officials were altered on 31 December 2019 to cases of pneumonia of unknown origins in Wuhan, there was a rapid response. Officials began to board all flights from Wuhan to check for passengers with symptoms of respiratory infection and isolated anyone so affected. By 5 January, surveillance was extended to include all passengers who had travelled from Wuhan in the previous 14 days. Anyone with symptoms was tested for 26 viruses including SARS, and was quarantined at home or in hospital. Using the national database of citizens plus the database of foreigners' entry cards, the Taiwanese authorities rapidly developed a sophisticated system that could provide immigration clearance for those travellers who presented minimal risk and formed a way of keeping track of and preventing the spread of the virus (Wang et al, 2020).

Australia also adopted a zero-COVID strategy at the start of the pandemic, closing its borders and even restricting the number of its own citizens who could return home. If a COVID-19 case did slip through the defences, there was meticulous contact-tracing to prevent major outbreaks (*The Economist*, 2021). The Australian CMO, Brendan Murphy, stated that the objective of the zero-COVID policy was to eliminate the virus: 'To be clear, we are not pursuing a path of "herd immunity", we are pursuing a path of control and suppression' (Grattan, 2020).

In West Africa, Senegal also adopted a rapid response approach. On 30 January, when the WHO declared COVID-19 an international emergency, the Senegalese started contingency planning (Shesgreen, 2020). When two individuals tested positive in March 2020, the president increased social distancing, imposed a curfew and restricted travel inside the country. At the same time, testing capacity was increased, aiming for test results within 24 hours. The government promised that every person who tested positive would get a treatment bed, reducing the risk that they would transmit the virus (Shesgreen, 2020).

Shifting framing of COVID-19 and changing policies: China and Japan

Not all countries in the western Pacific Rim framed COVID-19 as SARS-like. In China, the local authorities initially denied the existence of a new SARS-like disease. In December 2019, patients presenting at Wuhan hospitals with symptoms of COVID-19 were told they had flu or bronchitis (Honigsbaum, 2020, p. 262). When a whistle-blower, Dr Li Wenliang, posted online on 30 December 2019 that there were '7 SARS cases confirmed' at the seafood market, he was reprimanded by the local Security Office for 'illegal rumour mongering' and forced to sign a retraction (Honigsbaum, 2020, p. 262). However by 23 January 2020, hospitals in Wuhan were being overwhelmed by COVID-19 cases, and the authorities announced a lockdown.

Given the key role of the Chinese Communist Party in decision making and its lack of transparency, it can be difficult to follow the changing Chinese response to COVID-19. Wang and Mao (2021) have documented the reporting of COVID-19 in four Chinese papers. Following the Wuhan Health Committee's announcement on 31 December that there were cases of pneumonia of unknown origins, the newspapers began their coverage. From 1 January to 19 January, they published regular but limited reports. These reflected the official Party line that the new disease did not pose a particular danger and was controllable (Wang and Mao, 2021, p. 101). On 20 January, Nanshan Zhong, a national expert, announced that there was evidence of human-to-human transmission. There was an increase in the number of articles on COVID-19 as well as a new emphasis on the virus as a danger to people who were living in and around Wuhan. On 23 January, Chinese authorities announced a lockdown of Wuhan and the surrounding areas. There was a further increase in reporting, and a reframing of COVID-19 as a catastrophic event (Wang and Mao, 2021). Following this initial crisis lockdown in Wuhan, China adopted a zero-COVID policy, responding to new clusters of infections with blanket local lockdowns (Shepherd and Riordan, 2021).

In Japan the danger of COVID-19 was initially downplayed. This reflected the particular political circumstances: Prime Minister Shinzo Abe was coming to the end of his time in office, and the government wanted to avoid postponing the 2020 Olympics that Japan was due to host.

The Ministry of Health reported the first COVID-19 case on 15 January 2020 (*Japanese Times*, 2020). At this stage, the public health message from the ministry was one of reassurance. Media coverage referenced SARS, but the health ministry advised the public to take the same preventative measures that they would 'against a common cold or influenza' (*Japanese Times*, 2020). The Japanese government initiated Expert Meetings, which issued recommendations. The meeting on 9 March 2020 proposed a 'Japan Model' (Government of Japan, 2020, p. 5), involving identification of and rapid response to community clusters of infection, effective treatment with rapid diagnosis and intensive care treatment, and population behavioural change based on Japan's 3C policy: avoid closed spaces with poor ventilation, crowds and conversations in close proximity (Government of Japan, 2020, p. 2). Using backward contact tracing, Japanese researchers identified the role of superspreading events in the transmission of the virus (Lewis, 2020; Morelle, 2020).

Japan aspired to zero-COVID, but without the population database and advanced track and trace technology of Taiwan or the Chinese Communist Party's authoritarian control of the population, it was more an aspiration than reality (Shimzu et al, 2020).

Framing COVID-19 as seasonal flu; adopting a wait and see approach

The SARS and Ebola outbreaks were reported by the media in Europe and North America (Lewison, 2008), but they were events that mostly happened in other places and were relatively quickly forgotten.

In Europe and North America, seasonal influenza was more of an issue. Flu is highly contagious, spreads rapidly through the population and can be lethal, especially for older people and those with underlying health problems. Most years, levels of infection and deaths are limited and manageable; but on occasion, a new and more virulent strain emerges that bypasses the protection provided by vaccination. Such pandemics occurred in 1918–1919 (Spanish flu, H1N1), 1957 (Asian flu, H2N2) and 1968 (Hong Kong flu, H3N2) (Kilbourne, 2006). During the 1918–1919 pandemic, approximately 500 million people were infected and 50 million died (Jordan, 2019).

In Europe and North America, governments anticipated another flu pandemic. For example, Kilbourne (2006), reviewing the 20th-century flu pandemics, warned that 'the nature of the next pandemic virus cannot be predicted, but that it will arise from 1 of the 16 known HA [flu] subtypes in avian or mammalian species'.

In the UK, planning for a pandemic focused on influenza. Sally Davies, UK CMO (2010–2019), noted that the UK had had two emergency pandemic planning exercises, Winter Willow in 2007 and Cygnus in 2018, and these had identified shortcomings that had been rectified. Both were based on the assumption that the pandemic would be some sort of flu (Davies, 2020, Q727).

By the end of January 2020, there were clear warnings that a major epidemic was developing. By mid-January, researchers in China were publishing key information online, and this was picked up by researchers in Europe and North America. For example, in the UK modellers at Imperial College, London published their first predictions of the impact of the new virus on 17 January (Imai et al, 2020). It was clear that it represented a major danger when, on 23 January 2020, the Chinese authorities imposed a lockdown in Wuhan and on 30 January, the Director General of the WHO declared 'a public health emergency of international concern' (WHO, 2020a).

Countries in Europe and the Americas mainly disregarded these warnings and adopted a wait and see approach. In its review of response to the pandemic the WHO observed that February 2020 was the lost month because most countries failed to 'appreciate the threat' and adopted a 'wait and see' policy (2021, p. 29). Sally Davies, the former CMO, commenting on the UK response, noted that 'we were in groupthink. Our infectious disease experts really did not believe that SARS, or another SARS, would get from Asia to us. It is a form of British exceptionalism' (Davies, 2020, Q716).

Implicit in the wait and see approach was a herd immunity policy. Since it is extremely difficult to prevent flu viruses spreading, the accepted public health approach was to allow the virus to spread through the healthy population while seeking to protect high-risk groups, older people and those with underlying health problems. Eventually the epidemic would peter out as the population built up collective or 'herd' immunity. As Sally Davis noted, measures to control the spread of the virus measures tend to be ineffective against flu viruses: 'when you are planning for flu, the classic is you don't bother to test, so we didn't have a test-and-trace system to stand up. ... We would have to think differently if we had prepared for a SARS-type virus' (Davies, 2020, Q716).

In the US, the 'flu frame' also shaped the response to the virus. At the start of 2020, there was consensus among US policy makers that the virus was flu-like and not high risk. On 23 January, when the Chinese authorities announced a lockdown in the city of Wuhan, Trump was informed by his chief security briefer that the new disease was 'Just like flu. We don't think it's as deadly as SARS' (Woodward, 2020a, p. 230). This consensus shifted in March 2020 as the reality of the high level of infection and lethal nature of the disease became evident. In the summer of 2020, as the US presidential election approached, experts continued to emphasise the dangerous nature of COVID-19, but President Trump and his inner advisers returned to their initial framing. In September 2020, Trump argued that the virus would go away without a vaccine because 'You'll [the US population] develop like a herd mentality [immunity]. It's going to be herd-developed and that's gonna happen' (Mazza, 2020).

Abandoning the wait and see approach and replacing it with lockdown

As wait and see countries did not develop effective ways of interrupting the transmission of the virus, it rapidly became established as large-scale community transmission took place. The number of cases rose exponentially, as did hospital admissions and deaths, and there was a threat that both hospitals and mortuaries would be overwhelmed. The uncontrolled spread of the virus through wait and see countries can be traced through its impact on hospitals. In January 2020, a journalist in Wuhan described the impact of the virus: 'There are not enough hospitals and not enough beds, not enough doctors and not enough nurses, not enough rubber gloves and not enough face masks' (Fifield, 2020).

By late February, the virus was spreading rapidly in northern Italy. The general hospital in Cremona had 12 beds for patients with infectious disease. By 12 March 2020, it was treating 250 patients with COVID-19 (Harlan and Pitrelli, 2020).

In London, Northwick Park Hospital admitted its first suspected case of COVID-19 on 3 March 2020. Despite rapidly increasing the number of wards dedicated to COVID-19 patients by 19 March, the hospital was overwhelmed and could take no more cases (Mackintosh, 2020). The pandemic hit New York in early March 2020. At Wyckoff Heights Medical Center in Brooklyn, the first COVID-19 patient was admitted on 4 March, dying on 14 March (Shuster, 2020). The mortuary facilities in the hospital rapidly filled, and at night dead bodies were collected from the hospital and stored in refrigerated trailers that the city council had parked outside (Shuster, 2020). In Lima, Peru, the first case was recorded on 3 March. Initially, the spread was slow, with only 1,000 cases by the end of March; but then cases rose rapidly in April, as did the pressure on hospitals and mortuaries. At the Maria Auxiliadora hospital, the mortuary had a capacity for 6 bodies: between 13 and 16 bodies a day were stored on wards or in corridors. In addition, the hospital hired a 100-body freezer to store bodies before their cremation (Reuters, 2020).

To protect hospitals and to limit the rising death rates, most countries that had initially adopted a wait and see policy shifted to some form of lockdown, emergency measures to limit the spread of the virus by limiting social interactions. While there is no clear accepted definition of lockdown, Haider et al (2020) suggest the following definition: 'a set of measures aimed at reducing transmission of COVID-19 that are mandatory, applied indiscriminately to a general population and involve some restrictions on the established pattern of social and economic life' (2020, p. 2), such as school closures or a ban on all public transport. China initiated the first lockdown in Wuhan in January 2020 and by the end of March 2020, 32 of the 43 countries in Europe had locked down (BBC News, 2020h). (I will examine the shifting policies in the UK in more detail in Case Study 1.)

Effectiveness of the different frames

Johns Hopkins University in the US produced regular updates during the pandemic. Their data indicates that those territories nearest Wuhan that had the least time to react, used the SARS frame and adopted public health measures to prevent or limit the spread of the virus, had the lowest death rates (Johns Hopkins University, 2021, data from 27 September 2021). The Johns Hopkins data is based on the data reported by governments, and governments did not use the same criteria for reporting deaths. However the general trends are clear. Taiwan had a low number of deaths (841) and a low mortality rate, 3.55 per 100,000 population, and other countries in the western Pacific Rim were similarly low. South Korea had 2,450 deaths and 4.74 deaths per 100,000, Vietnam 18,400 deaths and 19.07 deaths per 100,000, Japan 17,475 deaths and 13.84 deaths per 100,000 and New Zealand 27 deaths and 0.55 deaths per 100,000. In contrast, countries that adopted the wait and see approach did far worse: Brazil had 594,200 deaths and 281.55 deaths per 100,000, the UK 136,465 deaths and 204.18 deaths per 100,000 and the US 687,746 and 209.53 deaths per 100,000.

Early 2021, vaccinations and the shifting policy context

The roll-out of effective COVID-19 vaccines in late 2020 changed the policy context. Countries that had the resources to purchase vaccines and had the logistics to deliver them started vaccinating and providing protection for their populations. The *New York Times* (2021) vaccination tracker estimated that by 12 August 2021 over 4.5 billion doses had been given, or 60 per 100 people globally. The distribution of these doses was uneven, with high-income countries, especially those with smaller populations, having the highest rates. The tracker showed that Malta had the highest rate of full vaccination, at 80 per cent of the population; the Gulf states, UAE (73 per cent), Bahrain

(65 per cent) and Qatar (65 per cent), also had high rates, as did countries in Europe and North America (eg, Iceland 71 per cent, Belgium 65 per cent, Canada 63 per cent, Denmark 62 per cent, UK 60 per cent, US 50 per cent). Low-income countries, especially in Africa and South America, had low rates of vaccination. The highest rate in sub-Saharan Africa was in Equatorial Guinea, where 9.7 per cent of the population was vaccinated.

Enabling herd immunity

For politicians, especially those in high-income countries such as the UK and US, vaccinations were considered to be the magic bullet, a technological fix offering a way out of the pandemic. In November 2020, Jonathan Van-Tam, the UK's Deputy CMO, announced that the preliminary clinical trial results of the Oxford/Astra Zeneca vaccine showed that 'this particular vaccine prevents disease' (Swinford, 2020). He observed that the vaccine was a huge milestone; that it and other vaccines could provide protection from COVID-19 and were a 'very important scientific breakthrough' (Swinford, 2020).

The rapid roll-out of COVID-19 vaccines enabled high-income countries that had abandoned herd immunity policies to reconsider them. For example, public health experts at Johns Hopkins University argued that herd immunity was an achievable goal but that in the case of COVID-19 it would mean that the virus would continue to circulate, However, because of the immunity built up through vaccination and infection, the effects would be minimal (D'Souza and Dowdy, 2021). In the UK, Matt Hancock, the minister responsible for overseeing vaccine development and roll-out observed that COVID-19 was 'an extraordinary challenge faced by the whole of humanity, science held out one great hope. And that hope is vaccination' (Hancock, 2021a). He stated that he had realised that 'a vaccine would be our way out the pandemic...' (Hancock, 2021a).

Blindsiding countries pursuing Zero-COVID policies

Countries in Europe and North America that had initially underestimated the threat were quick to exploit the benefits of vaccines. However, countries that adopted zero-COVID policies, with some exceptions (China with 56 per cent of the population fully vaccinated and Mongolia with 62 per cent), were far slower. For example, on 12 August 2021, 19 per cent of the population in Australia was fully vaccinated, 17 per cent in New Zealand, 16 per cent in South Korea and 2.7 per cent in Taiwan (*New York Times*, 2021).

While these countries continued to pursue zero-COVID policies, there were a number of factors that undermined their efforts (see Table 2.1). In Australia, there were tensions between federal and state politicians over zero-COVID policies. The Western Australia premier advocated maintaining a

Table 2.1: Factors undermining zero-COVID policies

Asymptomatic transmission	Unexplained cases identified following virus free periods.
Widespread transmission in other countries	Given the failure of many countries to control the spread of the virus and the emergence of new more contagious variants, there was a constant danger of the virus entering the country and the need for constant vigilance.
Political and population fatigue	While everyday life could continue as normal, the population had to adjust to some loss of liberty, for example periodic lockdowns when new cases were identified and restrictions on travel. Over time, these restrictions elicited resistance and political protests.
Lack of exit strategy	Given the relative success of zero-COVID policies, these countries were slow to develop vaccination programmes and offer a way out of the pandemic.

zero-COVID policy, while the federal prime minister indicated that this was absurd: 'once you get to 70% and 80% [of population vaccinated] at that level, and particularly at 80%, then you are managing the virus just like you would the flu' (Martin, 2021). This exchange took place when there was a lockdown in Sydney to control a major and uncontrolled outbreak of the Delta variant (Reuters, 2021).

In New Zealand on 17 August 2021, the Ministry of Health announced a move to Alert Level 4 (full lockdown) following the identification of a positive case, the first case of community transmission for six months (New Zealand Ministry of Health, 2021). In response to questions about the rapid lockdown, the New Zealand prime minister gave a one word answer, 'Australia', referring to the Sydney outbreak (McClure, 2021). The outbreak was a superspreading event with over 70 cases of the highly infectious Delta variant (Corlett, 2021). Chris Hipkins, the New Zealand minister for COVID-19 response observed that the event was a 'game changer', making existing protection look 'less adequate'. He argued that it raised 'some pretty big questions about what the long-term future of our plans are' and that at 'some point we will have to start to be more open in the future' (Corlett, 2021).

At the start of the pandemic, Hong Kong was one of the success stories. By rapidly shutting down its borders for eight months, it did not have a single COVID-19 case and residents could live a normal life. In March 2022, Hong Kong became a COVID-19 hotspot as the Omicron variant spread rapidly, overwhelming the public health protective measures. The death rate rose to 3.8 per 100,000 (in the UK, it had been 1.8 per 100,000 at its highest). With its high population density, Hong Kong had failed to develop a strategy for exiting zero-COVID. While it achieved good overall vaccination rates, with over 85 per cent of the population having at least one injection, it had failed to protect the most vulnerable. In the UK, more than 90 per cent of the over 65 population had two vaccinations and 80 per cent a booster. In Hong Kong, nearly 40 per cent of the over 80s were unvaccinated (Chivers, 2022).

Case Study 1: UK policy: from herd immunity to lockdowns and back again

Early March: herd immunity

In late January 2020, policy makers in the UK were alerted to the threat of COVID-19. On 24 January, the Civil Contingencies Committee (COBRA), which deals with major threats to national security, met to discuss COVID-19. The meeting was chaired by Matt Hancock, the Secretary of State for Health and Social Care, who later tweeted 'I have chaired a meeting of COBR on the response to Wuhan coronavirus. Official advice is that risk to the UK remains low' (Hancock, 2020a). On the same day, experts, including Richard Horton, editor of *The Lancet*, warned the government that the virus was a serious danger to public health in the UK (Calvert and Arbuthnott, 2021, p. 102). On 29 January, the UK had its first two confirmed cases of COVID-19: two Chinese nationals staying in a hotel in York. Despite the warning signals, the threat of COVID-19 did not initially attract much attention from policy makers.

When policy makers and their scientific advisers did discuss the risks of the new virus, they framed it as a type of seasonal flu (Syed, 2020). In an television interview on 5 March, Boris Johnson, the prime minister, outlined the options for responding to COVID-19, ranging from 'draconian' measures such as closing schools to 'to take it on the chin and take it all in one go and allow the disease to move through the population' (YouTube, 2020a). Given his belief that the virus was spreading slowly, 'not exponentially', Johnson favoured letting it spread.

In early March 2020, the UK government response to COVID-19 was one of minimalist intervention. On 3 March, the government adopted a Coronavirus Action Plan, based on the assumption that most people who were infected would have 'a mild-to-moderate, but self-limiting illness – similar to seasonal flu' (Farrar, 2022, p. 97). The core of the plan was to protect health services by slowing the spread of the virus. David Halpern, a member of the Scientific Advisory Group for Emergencies (SAGE), outlined the government strategy: 'to cocoon, to protect those at-risk groups so they don't catch the disease. By the time they come out of their cocooning, herd immunity has been achieved in the rest of the population' (Sengupta, 2020). On 13 March on BBC Radio 4, Sir Patrick Vallance, the Chief Scientific Adviser (CSA) stated: 'Our aim is to try and reduce the peak – not suppress it completely, also because most people get a mild illness, to build up some degree of herd immunity whilst protecting the most vulnerable' (Kermani, 2020).

Slamming on the lockdown brakes: late March 2020

By mid-March, it had become clear that the costs of treating COVID-19 as seasonal flu were too high. On 13 March, key policy makers, including Boris Johnson, Sir Patrick Vallance, Chris Whitty and Dominic Cummings, the prime minister's special adviser, held a meeting to review the government's strategy. The key points of the meeting were recorded on two whiteboards (Cummings 2021; Topping 2021). The first provided estimates of the likely outcomes of three policies or scenarios in terms of deaths and overwhelming of health services. In the first scenario, with no mitigation, there was a rapid rise in cases, with National Health Service (NHS) capacity rapidly exceeded and '100,000+ people dying in corridors' (Cummings, 2021). In the second scenario, the 'Current Plan', in which measures were taken to protect the vulnerable, the rise in cases was slower but the outcome was the same albeit spread over a longer time. In the third scenario, the new or 'Actual Plan', a lockdown of at least three weeks reduced the spread of the virus, allowing time for an 'NHS capacity ramp-up' so that it could cope.

The second whiteboard provided a more detailed analysis of the current policy (Plan A) and the proposed new policy (Plan B), the second and third scenarios. The board outlined the key policy issues:

- No vaccine in 2020
- Must avoid NHS collapse — + collapse is non linear, if happens, then not 1% but 2% die in R C W
- Our current 'plan' means 4k p/d [4,000 deaths per day] dying @peak
- Which means ... 2 weeks (?) before we catch up with Italy
- who do we not save? (emphasis in the original, Cummings, 2021).

The implication of the analysis were clear:

- To stop NHS collapse, we will probably have to 'lockdown'
- Lockdown = e/o [everyone] (except critical infrastructure people) stays home, pubs etc close
- who looks after people who can't survive alone?? (Cummings, 2021).

Those attending the meeting agreed that the costs of the current policy were too high and that to prevent 4,000 people a day dying and to prevent the NHS collapsing, the government had to lockdown all non-essential activities and movement. Given the prime minister's reluctance to act (Calvert and Arbuthnott, 2021, pp 194–220), the lockdown was delayed until 23 March.

Repeating the same mistakes

In the UK, excess deaths started to increase on 20 March and peaked on 17–24 April. Between 7 March and 8 May 2020, there were 47,243 excess deaths (Kontopantelis et al, 2021).

As the numbers of infections fell in May and the economic damage and costs of lockdown became more evident, pressure grew for the easing of restrictions. On 28 May, the prime minister announced there would be a major easing on 15 June, and non-essential shops could reopen. There was concern among public health experts that controls were being eased too quickly. On 23 June, SAGE expressed concern about the risk of accelerating transmission as too many restrictions were being eased at the same time and that local outbreaks were highly likely (SAGE, 2020a, minute 9).

Despite these concerns, the government adopted policies designed to increase economic activity, allowing travel to countries with high infection rates (Calvert and Arbuthnott, 2021, p. 335) and providing a subsidy for people to eat in the confined spaces of restaurants. By July, there was evidence that infection rates were on the rise again. By 6 August, SAGE was so concerned about the risk of a second wave that it warned the government that they would need to consider a short lockdown or 'circuit breaker' if infection rates continued to rise (SAGE, 2020b, minute 5).

Infection rates did indeed rise rapidly. By the start of October, there was evidence that a second wave was building rapidly. On 8 October, the SAGE committee noted infections were doubling every 8–16 days (SAGE, 2020c, minute 2, 10), and they called for a package of measures to halt the rise (SAGE, 2020c, minute 4). On 12 October, Boris Johnson made a speech in which he acknowledged the dangers of a new wave (Johnson, 2020a). However, he did not announce a national lockdown; instead he adopted a tiered system, with local restrictions linked to infection levels (Johnson, 2020a).

These measures did not work, and having resisted a circuit breaker lockdown, Boris Johnson (2020c) was forced to announce a lockdown in England on 31 October 2020 because hospitals were in danger of being overrun. This ran from 5 November 2020 until 3 December. The intention was to reopen the country for Christmas. On 16 December, Boris Johnson announced a relaxation of social distancing rules for Christmas. But with the rapid spread of the new Alpha variant and a resulting increase in hospital admissions and deaths, on 19 December, Johnson (2020d) was forced to announce a lockdown over the Christmas period in England, and the devolved administrations rapidly followed suit. The UK stayed effectively locked down until July 2021.

Finding a technological fix and learning to live with the virus

The second wave peaked in mid-January 2020, with a rolling daily average of 60,000 new cases, 40,000 COVID-19 patients in hospital and an average daily COVID-related death toll of 1,200 (COBR, 2021). By 22 February, the social distancing measures had had a major impact on the second wave; the rolling average of new daily cases had fallen to 11,187 and the daily average of COVID-related deaths had fallen to 480 (COBR, 2021). At a Downing Street press conference, Boris Johnson announced a four-step road map for easing lockdown restrictions as long as there was successful and effective deployment of vaccinations, hospitals were not overwhelmed and the risk assessment was not changed by a new variant (Johnson, 2021a).

The fourth and final step of the road map, including the removal of all legal limits on social contacts, was due on 21 June. The first three steps took place on the indicated dates. However, on 14 June, Johnson (2021b) announced that Step 4 would be delayed as the Delta variant was driving up both infections (8,000 cases a day and increasing by 64 per cent a week) and hospitalisations (rising by 50 per cent a week). He stressed that a delay would provide time for all over 50s and vulnerable people to be offered full vaccination (Johnson, 2021b).

On 12 July, Boris Johnson (2021c) announced that despite the spread of the Delta variant, the rising number of cases, rising hospitalisations and rising death rates, all legal limits on social contacts in England would be lifted on 19 July. There was concern in the scientific community (Sample, 2021). In a speech on 19 July, Johnson justified his decision, arguing that a further delay would 'simply delay the inevitable' and that the issue was 'if not now, when?' (Johnson 2021d). He noted that hospitalisations and deaths would increase, but that such increases were within 'the margins of what our scientists predicted at the outset of the roadmap' (Johnson 2021d), and by implication, acceptable risks.

On the same day, Nadhim Zahawi (2021), the government's vaccine minister, observed that there was no perfect time to end lockdown but that the vaccination programme had provided protection for UK residents and substantially reduced the rate of hospitalisation. There were uncertainties as new mutations could undermine the immunity provided by the vaccine: 'coronavirus mutates, just like flu, we must stay one step ahead of the virus' (Zahawi, 2021). He argued that 'As we [the UK population] learn to live with COVID-19 we must be pragmatic about how we manage the risks we face' (Zahawi, 2021).

By the end of August 2021, it was possible to identify the risks that the UK government considered acceptable. Data for 25 August (Gov.UK, 2021a) indicated that the number of cases was rising, with 35,847 new cases per day (236,796 in that week); 859 people had been admitted to hospital (6,172 in the week); 147 people had died who tested positive (743 in the week). While the UK government did not formally state what it was willing to tolerate to maintain current policies, newspaper reports (denied by the Prime Minister's Office) indicated that the prime minister would only impose a further lockdown if deaths exceeded 1,000 a week (Parsley, 2021).

In February 2022, the UK prime minister removed all public health measures to control the spread of COVID-19, and did not reimpose them when in April 2022 infection rates reached record levels. Government data indicated that in the week to 6 April 2022, 389,368 people tested positive, 16,478 were admitted to hospital and 1,194 died having tested positive in the previous 28 days (Gov.UK, 2022a).

A number of factors explain this normalisation of COVID-19 infection:

- Politics: Although Boris Johnson as UK prime minister did not face an election until 2024, in early 2022 his position was becoming increasingly precarious because of Partygate – media reports of parties held at his official residence during lockdowns. (He was forced to resign in July 2022.) In January 2022, the Metropolitan Police decided to investigate 12 events, including at least three attended by Johnson. Focusing on removing restrictions offered a popular distraction.
- Less lethal variants: As a short piece of genetic material, SARS-CoV-2 mutated rapidly, and some mutations had genetic advantages (usually of transmissibility) that enabled them to spread rapidly and become the dominant variant. The virus has evolved and in England, the original Wuhan virus was replaced first by the Alpha variant, then the Delta variant, followed by the Omicron variant which in turn was replaced by its mutations, initially BA.2 and then in June 2022 BA.4 and BA5. Each variant tended to be more transmissible. With Omicron there was a marked decline in lethalness. At its peak in January 2022, the Omicron variant caused over a million infections a day in England; at its peak in January 2021 the Alpha variant infected less than 400,000 people a day (Spencer and Lintern, 2022, p. 12). Despite Omicron's high rate of infection there were fewer deaths: 8,100 deaths in January 2022 compared with 16,528 COVID-related deaths in February 2021 (Gov.UK, 2022b).
- Vaccination: Vaccinated people could still be infected by the virus, but vaccination tended to reduce the severity of the illness, so while admissions to hospital increased, there were fewer severely ill COVID-19 patents requiring intensive care unit (ICU) beds or ventilators. The pressure on hospitals increased, but most were able to continue operating normally

(Barnes and Neville, 2022). Hospital staff had learnt from the previous waves and were able to adjust to the new wave (see Chapter 6).

- Public acceptance of reduced precaution: In a number of countries there were high-profile protests against COVID-19 restrictions in early 2022. The freedom convoy demonstrations in Canada stimulated violent protests in France and the Netherlands (Associated Press, 2022). Taking precautions that visibly change a person's appearance highlights the dangers and undermines their sense of normality. As Harries noted in his analysis of why individuals living in areas of high flood risk did not take precautions, 'people sometimes put what Giddens [1991] calls their ontological security above their physical security' (Harries, 2008, p. 479).
- Policy makers' perception that the population was developing herd immunity: The 'Government expects that the population's defences against new variants will continue to strengthen as immunity increases through advances in vaccine technology and repeated exposure to the virus' (HM Government, 2022, p. 8).
- Media attention had moved on: When on 24 February 2022, the Russian Federation invaded the Ukraine, media attention shifted to the war, and COVID-19 lost its status as the lead story.

Comment

Framing provides a way to identify the key features of a novel situation. A frame does not provide a comprehensive picture, but rather it highlights key features of the situation. The effectiveness of this device depends on how well it captures the salient features of reality. Both the SARS frame and the flu frame captured some but not all the key features of COVID-19. Like SARS, COVID-19 is a highly contagious virus facilitating superspreader events. Most COVID-19 variants directly affect the respiratory system, causing pneumonia, and this can result in serious illness and death (Crawford, 2021, Table 5). Given these similarities, it was reasonable to adopt the same preventive measures that had worked effectively against SARS and to aim for the elimination of the virus.

Like seasonal flu, COVID-19 is a highly contagious virus, and like flu it can cause serious illness and death, but most people only have a mild illness – with serious illness and death mainly affecting vulnerable groups (Crawford, 2021, Table 5). It did not seem unreasonable to treat the new coronavirus as flu-like and to adopt the same approach, that is, to mitigate the effects of the virus by protecting the vulnerable, while allowing the virus to spread among the young and healthy, creating collective or herd immunity.

There were important features of COVID-19 that neither frame captured and this created cognitive dissonance, a significant difference between the predictions based on the frames and what actually happened – or, as Barack

Obama, a former US president put it, 'the classic example of reality biting back' (Obama, 2020). The most obvious difference was the speed at which and ways in which the new coronavirus was transmitted. When researchers (Cepelewicz, 2021) initially tried to predict the spread of SARS-CoV-2, many used data from the SARS epidemic, but the new virus spread twice as fast as SARS and much of the transmission was hidden by presymptomatic and asymptomatic transmission (Cepelewicz, 2021).

While flu can be spread through presymptomatic and asymptomatic transmission, such spread is more limited. SARS-CoV-2 is more contagious. It spreads more rapidly and has a greater propensity to superspreader events (CDC, 2021a). SARS-CoV-2 is also more lethal than seasonal flu: early case fatality rates were at least 1 death per 100 cases, which, as Farrar notes, is ten times more lethal than seasonal flu (Farrar, 2022, p. 98). Given the very limited testing at the start of the pandemic, countries that adopted the flu frame and a wait and see strategy underestimated its spread, and were forced to react when rising infections and hospital admissions threatened to overwhelm their health services. In the UK, the whiteboard photograph taken on 13 June provides a clear pictorial record of policy makers acknowledging an unanticipated reality and shifting their policy to suppressing the virus by lockdown. However, they did not abandon their belief that COVID-19 could be converted into and managed as if it were flu. The development of effective COVID-19 vaccines provided them with a way of pursuing herd immunity policies without overwhelming health services or creating an unacceptable body count.

Countries that adopted zero-COVID policies were relatively successful at eliminating the virus at the start of the pandemic. However, as the pandemic progressed, so they faced challenges. Some of these were created by the nature of COVID-19. Its asymptomatic and superspreading qualities meant that after months of no cases, community clusters could suddenly flare up, requiring reimposition of control measures. Other challenges came from the external environment. As other countries failed to eliminate the virus and sustained community transmission, so new, more virulent variants evolved. To protect themselves, zero-COVID countries had to maintain strict controls especially over international travel, and found it difficult to develop an exit strategy.

3

The risks of COVID-19: probability, categorisation and outcomes

Risk: probability and outcome

One way of thinking about risk is in terms of the probability of one or more outcomes. Probability provides a way of using knowledge derived from the observation of past events to predict the likelihood of similar outcomes in the future. There is a strong technical and objective reality to probability; it is often expressed numerically. In contrast, outcomes are more subjective and relate to personal and collective values.

This difference can be seen in gambling. When individuals choose to bet on a horse race, they are taking a risk. If their horse loses, they lose their stake, but if their horse wins, they win. The size of their winnings depends on the horse's 'odds', that is, the probability of the horse winning based mainly on evidence from previous races. The choices individuals make depend on their personal preferences and values. If they value certainty, they will not bet. This means that they can be sure they will not lose money, but they will forego the chance of winning and the excitement of betting. If they value risk-taking and the chance to make a big win, then they will back a 'long shot'.

When choices are made on behalf of others and the outcomes affect different social groups, it is no longer just a matter of personal preference but one of collective values. This can be seen in the process of triaging, a way of prioritising and allocating scarce resources, for example following a battle or disaster or in hospital accident and emergency units.

Triaging was developed during the Napoleonic Wars (1803–1815) by the French military surgeon Dominique Jean Larrey to minimise deaths (Skandalakis et al, 2006). In the battlefield setting, it involves categorising the injured and allocating resources between three main risk categories:

Category 1 No active treatment for the most seriously injured (low probability of survival);
Category 2 Immediate treatment for the seriously injured (good chance of survival with treatment);
Category 3 Delayed treatment for those who have minor injuries (near certainty of survival).

Larrey observed that: 'those dangerously wounded must be attended first entirely *without regard to rank or distinction* and those less severely wounded must wait until the gravely hurt have been operated and addressed' (emphasis added, Skandalakis et al, 2006, p. 1396). Triaging represented a shift from allocating resources on the basis of social status to one based on collective benefit.

During the COVID-19 pandemic, health resources were not adequate to meet the demands and collective choices had to be made. In this chapter, I examine how these choices were made and what these choices tell us about social values.

COVID-19: identifying at-risk individuals

In contemporary societies, one of the key roles of government is to protect its citizens from preventable illness and death. In countries that adopted a zero-COVID approach, such protection centred on preventing the transmission of the virus. In countries, that adopted a wait and see policy, allowing the virus to get a foothold, governments initially identified and advised the most at-risk individuals to protect themselves, but when they had to move to lockdown policies then the whole population became a COVID-19 risk/disease population (Aronowitz, 2009), categorised according to the risk of serious illness and death.

The emerging evidence

Viruses that infect the respiratory system tend to affect most severely older people and people with underlying health conditions, and they are more likely to be hospitalised and die if they are infected (Glezen et al, 2000). By February 2020, epidemiological evidence was emerging from China that these individuals were at risk if they were infected by SARS-CoV-2. The Chinese Coronavirus Epidemiology Team (Novel Coronavirus Pneumonia Emergency Response Epidemiology Team, 2020) analysed the first 72,314 Chinese cases of COVID-19 with 44,672 confirmed cases. They reported on the:

- Severity of the illness: Most reported cases were mild; indeed, 889 cases (1.2 per cent) were asymptomatic. However, 2,087 (4.7 per cent of confirmed cases) were critical – with respiratory failure, septic shock, and/or multiple organ dysfunction/failure – and 1,023 died (a case fatality rate of 2.3 per 100).
- Impact of age: Children and young people could be infected (there were 965 cases aged 0–19) but they were unlikely to become seriously ill. Older people had more serious illness. Among the 1,408 cases aged over 80, there were 208 (14.8 per hundred cases) deaths.

- Impact of pre-existing illnesses that increased the probability of severe illness: Individuals who had no underlying illness had a 0.9 per cent case fatality rate; this increased to 5.6 per cent for patients with cancer, 6 per cent with hypertension, 6.3 per cent with chronic respiratory disease, 7.3 per cent with diabetes and 10.5 per cent with cardiovascular disease.
- Impact of gender: Men were more vulnerable (2.8 per cent case fatality) than women (1.7 per cent).

Similar epidemiological evidence was collected later in the pandemic in other countries. In the US, the CDC monitored deaths. Their analysis of deaths up to 3 October 2020 indicated an excess death rate of 299,028 of which 198,081 could be directly attributed to COVID-19 (Rossen et al, 2020). The overall excess death rate was five times higher than the average annual death rate from seasonal flu. The increase in deaths was most marked among older people and among minority ethnic groups, especially Hispanics.

Risk categorisation

As the virus spread through Europe and North America in March 2020, and governments shifted to lockdown, so they issued guidance on the risk that the virus represented to different groups in the population and how they should mitigate this risk. Table 3.1 summarises the categorisation in the UK, the US and Canada in the early stages of the pandemic (May 2020). In each country the population was divided into three risk categories:

- Individuals with a low risk of a poor outcome if infected; the majority of the population. These individuals were advised to protect themselves by increased social distancing.
- Individuals with an increased risk of a poor outcome, such as older people and those with specific underlying health problems. They were advised to take extra precautions.
- Individuals with the highest risk of a poor outcome, especially those with compromised immune systems. They were advised to self-isolate and shield themselves by avoiding all social contact except for essential medical care.

This risk categorisation enabled policy makers to communicate to the public the different levels of risk and the types of actions that individuals should take to mitigate such risk. The categorisation differed in detail. In the US, the CDC's categorisation was more fine-grained than that in the UK and Canada. For example, the CDC drew attention to the increased risk for people with disabilities, people experiencing homelessness, and racial and

Table 3.1: Official categorisation of risk groups and lockdown advice in May 2020

	UK	US	Canada
Low risk	Younger, fitter, healthy individuals – stay or work at home if possible, maintain social distance when out	Younger, fitter, healthy individuals living in the community – wash hands, avoid close social contact, wear a face mask, cover coughs and sneezes, and disinfect surfaces	All Canadians except those with risk factors – reduce social contacts by social distancing maintaining at least 2m distance outside household, minimise travel, avoid crowds
Intermediate/ high risk	Over 70s, those eligible for annual flu vaccination, pregnant women – socially isolate and do not go out if possible	Pregnant women, people with disabilities, homeless people and racial and ethnic minority groups – social distance, hand wash, cover coughs and sneezes, clean surfaces and launder safely	Pregnant women – stay at home as much as possible, avoid unnecessary visitors to home, shift interactions with health professionals to phone or videoconferencing
Highest risk	Clinically extremely vulnerable (who have received a warning letter from the NHS) – shield, no social contact except for essential medical care	Over 65s, people living in nursing homes and long-term care facilities, people with underlying health problems – protective measures plus minimisation of social contacts	Over 65s, people with compromised immune systems and/ or underlying health conditions – self-isolate and avoid all social contacts outside household

Source: UK (Cabinet Office, 2020), US (CDC, 2020a) and Canada (Government of Canada, 2020)

ethnic minority groups, and stressed the vulnerability of those living in a nursing home or long-term care facility.

Policy makers in different countries were selective in the ways in which they used the evidence, excluding some at-risk groups and including others for which there was no evidence of increased risk:

- The exclusion of people from Black and minority ethnic (BAME) groups from the high-risk category in the UK. While BAME groups were proportionally smaller in the UK than the US, they were still substantial and had a higher incidence of underlying health problems such as diabetes. Many were front-line workers in health, social care and transport.
- The exclusion of front-line workers from the high-risk category. Governments excluded such workers as they needed them to continue operating in hazardous settings.

- The inclusion of pregnant women in the high-risk category. Pregnant women were included in this category despite there being no evidence that they were more vulnerable than other women of their age.

Risk categorisation and social values

While the virus could infect individuals of all ages, the epidemiological data indicated that younger age groups, especially children and young adults, were most likely to be infected and to transmit the virus. Older people were less likely to be infected, but if this happened they were more likely to become seriously ill and die. This could clearly be seen in the data for California (California Department of Public Health, 2021). In California, 78.6 per cent of the population was younger than 60 and accounted for 84.7 per cent of COVID-19 cases, but only 36.4 per cent of deaths. Individuals aged over 80 accounted for 3.9 per cent of the population, 2.7 per cent of recorded cases and 38.2 per cent of all COVID-related deaths.

Herd immunity: valuing the generations

At the start of the pandemic, several countries in Europe and North America explored the strategy of herd immunity, allowing the virus to spread among younger people who had less risk of developing severe COVID-19, thereby developing population or herd immunity. This strategy was most explicitly outlined in the Great Barrington Declaration (2020), an online international petition. The Declaration noted that children and young adults had a low risk of serious illness stating that 'Indeed, for children, COVID-19 is less dangerous than many other harms, including influenza' (Great Barrington Declaration, 2020). The Declaration argued that 'The most compassionate approach that balances the risks and benefits of reaching herd immunity, is to allow those who are at minimal risk of death to live their lives normally to build up immunity to the virus through natural infection' (Great Barrington Declaration, 2020). The Declaration argued that older people who were at highest risk should be shielded from the virus by 'Focused Protection'. The measures needed for such protection were not specified.

While no country has publicly committed to a herd immunity policy, it is clear that some experimented with this approach. Sweden perhaps went the furthest. At the start of the pandemic, policy makers there decided not to introduce legally enforceable public health measures to control the spread of the virus (Bjorklund and Ewing, 2020). There was no extensive use of track and trace and no early lockdown. The government did not pass laws to limit crowds on public transport, in shopping malls or other public spaces (Claeson and Hanson, 2021). The architect of the policy, Anders Tegnell, an epidemiologist in the Public Health Agency, commended a proposal 'to keep schools open to reach herd immunity faster'. When Mika Salminen, his counterpart in the Finnish Health Agency, decided not to keep schools in Finland open, as 'over time children are still going to spread the infection to other are age groups' and closing schools would reduce 'the attack rate of the disease on the elderly' by 10 per cent, Tegnell suggested that '10 percent might be worth it?' (Bjorklund and Ewing, 2020). Daycare and schools remained open in Sweden in 2020.

The implicit values underpinning the Swedish herd immunity strategy were that fitter and younger people should be allowed to continue with their economic, educational and social activities, even if this meant that some older and other more vulnerable people died.

Before lockdown on 23 March 2020, the UK adopted a wait and see approach based on an implicit herd immunity strategy. While it was in operation, journalists and others were able to elicit explicit statements of the values underpinning policy, mainly from sources that wanted to remain anonymous. There were parallels with Sweden, with policy makers being willing to tolerate (a degree of) serious illness and death among the elderly to enable normal life to continue for the rest of the population. One source told *Sunday Times* journalists: 'It's the intergenerational question. It is unsustainable to have people in their youth put their whole life on hold for months while the economy tanks to save a 91-year-old who would have died six months later anyway' (Shipman and Wheeler, 2020). Policy makers were unwilling to own such values in public. For example, the *Sunday Times* reported that Dominic Cummings had justified herd immunity policy, saying that 'if that means some pensioners die, too bad' (Shipman and Wheeler, 2020). This was immediately denied by the Prime Minister's Office (Smyth, 2020). There was some epidemiological evidence that significant events such as outbreaks of infectious disease and heatwaves impacted disproportionately on vulnerable individuals in the short term resulting in a short-term increase in death rates followed by a period of reduced mortality, so overall deaths averaged out (ONS, 2019). However, no policy maker in the UK was willing to use this argument in public to justify a herd immunity policy.

Protecting hospitals: sacrificing older people

Countries that adopted a wait and see approach at the start of the pandemic allowed the virus to spread rapidly. As testing facilities were initially limited, the first sign that the virus had established a foothold was a rapid rise in hospital admissions, followed a few weeks later by a rapid rise in the number of people dying. These rises meant that hospitals came under severe pressure and in some cases were overwhelmed, having to turn away patients (I discuss this in more detail in Chapter 6).

The phenomenon of hospitals being overwhelmed was first observed in Wuhan in late January and resulted in a lockdown (Fifield, 2020), then in Northern Italy in late February (Harlan and Pitrelli, 2020) and then more widely across Europe and North America in March 2020.

As I show in Chapter 5, hospitals generally reacted rapidly to the threat of being overwhelmed, and concentrated resources on younger fitter individuals who were more likely to survive.

In Northern Italy, the sudden surge of COVID-19 patients in late February 2020 meant that hospitals ran out of beds, especially those in ICUs that had facilities for ventilating patients. They had to prioritise patients with the best chance of survival. As Antonio Presenti, the head of Lombardy's intensive crisis care unit, put it: 'It's as if you were asking what to do if an atomic bomb explodes. ... You declare defeat. We'll try to salvage what is salvageable' (Harlan and Pitrelli, 2020).

In the UK, infection rates rose rapidly in March 2020 and hospitals in London were the first to come under pressure. On 11 March, Northwick Park Hospital, near Heathrow Airport, reported a doubling of COVID-19 admissions in two days (Mackintosh, 2020). On 19 March, senior hospital staff declared an emergency, closing the hospital to new admissions. The British Medical Association (BMA), the UK's doctors' professional association, responded to the rapidly increasing demand for services by issuing guidance to its members on how they should ration services. The BMA recommended triaging so that 'younger, healthier people [are] given priority over older people and ... those with an underlying illness...' (Campbell et al, 2020).

At the same Chris Whitty, England's CMO, examined ways of developing an 'ethical' tool to help doctors prioritise the use of intensive care facilities (Insight, 2020). On 20 March, the Moral and Ethical Advisory Group met to discuss the issue (Calvert and Arbuthnott, 2021, p. 211). The committee's chair, Sir Jonathan Montgomery, offered to provide guidance, and one of his colleagues, Mark Griffiths, produced a triage tool that categorised and scored patients on three criteria: age, clinical frailty and comorbidity (see Table 3.2). Patients who scored 8 or under were categorised as being eligible for the most intensive treatment (ICU-based care). Patients who scored over 8 were not considered to be eligible for intensive treatment in an ICU, but could receive 'ward-based care'. There was a third category, 'patients not normally for full active management'. This category seems to have been made up of individuals who were very severely frail, 'typically they could not recover from even a minor illness', and those who were terminally ill and likely to die within six months. They were considered suitable for domiciliary care with the provision of face mask oxygen, if necessary. This decision tool provided the basis of triaging, enabling resources to be directed to those who had the best chance of survival. However, such triaging targeted resources

Table 3.2: COVID-19 Decision Support Tool

Age	Points	Clinical Frailty Scale	Points	Co-morbidity	Points
Under 50	0	Very fit	1	Cardiac arrest in last three years	2
50–60	1	Well	2	Chronic condition, 3+ hospital admissions in last year	2
61–65	2	Managing well	3	Chronic condition, 4+ weeks for current in-patient	2
66–70	3	Vulnerable	4	Congestive heart failure	1
71–75	4	Mildly frail	5	Hypertension	1
76–80	5	Moderately frail	6	Severe/irreversible neurological condition including dementia	1
Over 80	6	Severely frail	7	Chronic liver disease	1
		Very severely frail	8	End-stage renal failure	1
		Terminally ill	9	Diabetes	1
				Uncontrolled or active malignancy	1

Note: The precise scoring of the Clinical Frailty Scale is not clear and women were allocated -1
Source: Financial Times (2020)

at younger healthier individuals, effectively denying older people, especially those with some frailty or underlying health problems, access to intensive care. Given the sensitivity of such value judgements, they provoked hostile media commentary. Although the version of the document published in the media carried the NHS logo (*Financial Times*, 2020), policy makers denied its existence and distanced themselves from it. For example, the National Institute for Health Care and Excellence (NICE) tweeted that it had not developed or endorsed the tool (NICE, 2020). Despite such formal denials, it appears that a version of the document were distributed in the NHS and used to inform decision making (Insight, 2020).

The care home disaster

In the first wave of the pandemic in high-income countries, older people living in residential facilities were particularly vulnerable, with a disproportionate number being infected and dying. In a review of evidence, Taylor (2020) finds that in 26 high-income countries, 'elder-care home residents have accounted for 47 per cent of recorded coronavirus deaths', with Canada, where 80 per cent of COVID-19 deaths took place in care homes, topping the list.

The Canadian Institute for Health Information (2021) investigated the high death rate in Canada. After death rates in the first two waves (1 March 2020 to 30 June and 1 September 2020 to 15 February 2021) were examined, it was found that they did not improve; indeed, in the second wave there were more outbreaks in care homes and a higher death rate (Canadian Institute for Health Information, 2021, p. 4). Up to 15 February 2021, 14,000 residents of care homes had died and 30 staff, while approximately 69 per cent of all COVID-19 deaths were in care homes. The institute attributed the high rates to the poor quality services, low staffing levels, poor infection control and lack of personal protective equipment (PPE) (Canadian Institute for Health Information, 2021, p. 22). These were combined with fewer physician visits, fewer transfers of residents to hospital for care and a general lack of support from the wider health-care system (Canadian Institute for Health Information, 2021, pp 15–16).

In the UK, there was a similar failure to protect care home residents. The *Sunday Times* Insight Team calculated that during the first six months of the pandemic there were 59,000 excess deaths, of which 25,000 were in care homes (Insight, 2020, p. 7).

The main driver of care home infection in the UK was the discharge of patients from hospital. At the start of the pandemic, patients were discharged to care homes without having COVID-19 tests. The Public Accounts Committee examined the impact of government policies on the care sector and concluded that, while the NHS had coped with the first wave of the virus, it had partly done so at the cost of the care sector. The committee observed that:

> **Discharging patients from hospital into social care without first testing them for COVID-19 was an appalling error.** Shockingly, Government policy up to and including 15 April was to not test all patients discharged from hospital for COVID-19. … Belatedly, after discharging 25,000 people from hospitals to care homes between 17 March and 15 April, the Department confirmed a new policy of testing everyone prior to admission to care homes. (Emphasis in the original, House of Commons, Public Accounts Committee, 2020, Conclusions and Recommendations, para 2)

Comment

While older people were categorised as being at risk if they contracted COVID-19, the precise significance of such categorisation and the values implicit in decisions based on such categorisation changed with the changing policy context. When governments adopted wait and see policies, they prioritised maintaining normal life for younger healthier people over protecting older and other vulnerable people. As it became evident that hospitals were being overwhelmed, most countries adopted emergency lockdown measures. Such measures reflected changed priorities and values, a willingness to disrupt the normal lives and activities of younger healthier people to protect older and other vulnerable people. However, while such lockdowns reduced the rates of infection and provided protection for older people over time, at the peak of each wave before the measures started to work, the emergency measure taken to protect hospitals and their intensive support units, such as triaging patients and, in the UK, discharging older people to care homes without COVID-19 tests, disadvantaged older people.

Case Study 2: Pregnant women and the precautionary principle

In this case study, I consider the special case of pregnant women, who in the UK, US and Canada were categorised as at risk. This categorisation was based on the precautionary principle, focusing on the value of a possible outcome rather than its probability: a 'better safe than sorry' strategy.

The evidence

At the time pregnant women were first classified as being at risk, there was no evidence supporting such a classification, as the UK's CMO, Chris Whitty, observed: 'Infections and pregnancy are not a good combination in general and that is why we have taken the very precautionary measure, whilst we find out more' (Rev, 2020a).

Emerging evidence at the start of the pandemic indicated that pregnant women did not have an increased probability of serious illness or that their unborn babies were at-risk. In the UK, a national prospective observational cohort study based on data from the UK Obstetric Surveillance System was published on 8 June 2020 (Knight et al, 2020). Data for 1 March to 14 April indicated that 427 pregnant women were admitted to hospital with COVID-19. The women in the study had similar rates of admission to critical care units and mortality to those of other women of reproductive age. There was some evidence that a small group of babies (2 per cent) might be infected, but generally the outcomes were reassuring. Matar and colleagues (2020) reviewed 24 studies mainly from China. They concluded that pregnant women in these studies had similar clinical characteristics and outcomes to their non-pregnant peers, and there was little evidence that they infected their unborn babies. However, compared with non-infected pregnant women, they were more likely to have a Caesarean section and a premature birth (Matar et al, 2020).

Evidence from later in the pandemic indicated that the virus did represent a threat to pregnant women and their unborn babies. In the US, the CDC reviewed the evidence, and concluded that while the overall risk of severe illness was low, pregnant women had an increased risk of severe illness if infected by the virus over non-pregnant women (CDC, 2021a). Such risks were increased by underlying medical conditions and by age. Pregnant women were also at risk of premature birth and other birth complications (CDC, 2021a).

Among the articles that the CDC cited as their sources of evidence was a systematic review conducted by Wei and colleagues (2021). This included 42 studies that examined the impact of COVID-19 on pregnancy. While both asymptomatic infection and mild illness had an impact on pregnant women and the outcome of pregnancy, the most marked impact was with severe COVID-19 illness, which was associated with pre-eclampsia, pre-term birth and still-birth, gestational diabetes, ICU admission, mechanical ventilation, caesarean delivery and low birth weight (Wei et al, 2021).

At the start of the pandemic, there was no evidence that COVID-19 infection presented a particular threat to pregnant women and their unborn babies. Public health experts included them in a high or at-risk category as a precautionary measure. Over time, evidence has emerged that justified this categorisation.

Has high-risk categorisation protected or helped pregnant women?

Despite categorising pregnant women as at risk, governments have taken little action to protect these women beyond warning them of the risks and advising them to be careful. For example, the CDC issued the following advice:

> It is especially important for pregnant and recently pregnant people, and those who live or visit with them, to take steps to protect themselves and others from getting COVID-19. Limit in-person interactions with people who might have been exposed to COVID-19… and get a COVID-19 vaccine as soon as you can. (CDC, 2021b)

Having identified the danger, the CDC was passing the responsibility for protection to the women themselves.

The impact of pandemics on women

Despite the CDC using the non-gendered term pregnant people (CDC, 2021b), they are biologically women, and as such experience the threats and dangers associated with their sex together with those relating to pregnancy.

In previous epidemics, measures taken to stop the spread of viruses, such as lockdowns, increased the vulnerability of women to the hazards of everyday life, such as sexual exploitation and mental health issues. During the Ebola epidemic in 2014–2016, the lockdown measures in Sierra Leone increased the vulnerability of women. There was a sharp increase in pregnancies, especially among teenage girls, reflecting increased sexual violence and the sale of sex to pay for essentials (Whyte, 2016). This in turn was linked to increased mortality from illicit abortions (Mitchell, 2017) and an increase in maternal complications, deaths and infant deaths in a country that already had the highest rates in the world. Elston et al (2020) found that there was systematic under-reporting of maternal deaths especially in rural areas, as in many villages here was no way of registering deaths and many health-care workers were reluctant to register them. They noted that most women wanted to give birth in a medical facility, but there were barriers that many women especially in rural areas could not overcome. They observed that the epidemic heightened these barriers, increasing mortality and complications. Pregnant women were active agents in managing their pregnancies, but to do this they had to balance and deal with a variety of risks: 'a woman's choice to deliver in the village is not a result of passive inaction or lack of knowledge about the potential risks she may face, but rather an active choice to reduce risks that she perceives as being of more importance' (Elston et al, 2020 p. 87).

Emerging evidence from the COVID-19 pandemic indicates that in high-income countries the general measures taken to control COVID-19 increased women's vulnerability, especially impacting on their mental health. In a study of 40 mid-life women living through lockdown in South Australia, Ward and his colleagues (2022) found that they experienced uncertainty and fear caused by the uncertain aetiology of the virus, the threat of illness, the lockdowns and disruption of their future. To counter such uncertainty, the women searched for areas that they could control, and developed strategies to create a sense of control and normality – thereby reducing their anxieties about the perceived chaos of events (Ward et al, 2022).

Pregnant women in the pandemic

For pregnant women, the challenges and risks of the pandemic were exacerbated by their pregnancy. This is particularly reflected in studies of their mental health.

In a web-based survey of 403 pregnant women in Turkey, Sut and Kucukkaya (2020) found that 64.5 per cent reported being anxious and 56.3 per cent depressed. These findings were in line with other studies during the pandemic that reported rates of between 63 per cent and 68 per cent compared with pre-pandemic rates of 22.3 per cent and less. Lebela and colleagues' (2020) online survey of 1,987 pregnant women in Canada noted that anxiety and depression typically affected 10 and 25 per cent of pregnant women, but during the pandemic those reporting anxiety rose to 37 per cent and depression to 57 per cent.

Lebela and colleagues (2020) found that women worried both about the COVID-19 threat to their own life and to their unborn babies. But these anxieties were compounded by other risks. Women reported a decline in general health-care support and support for their pregnancy (74 per cent reported problems accessing health care) and were concerned about not receiving adequate support. Most participants (89 per cent) reported changes in pre-natal care with cancelled appointments (36 per cent) and not being able to bring a support person (90 per cent). The direct threat of COVID-19 and the decline of health-care support were compounded by other challenges, including strained relationships with partners and declining contacts outside households: 18.3 per cent of the participants stopped working, and social isolation was rated a greater worry than the direct threat of COVID-19 (Lebela et al, 2020, pp 7–8).

In the UK and Belgium, pregnant women also experienced increased anxiety and isolation during the pandemic, as well as reduced access to a variety of services. Aptaclub's (2020) UK survey of 100 pregnant women and women with young babies (aged 0–4 months) found that nearly half of those surveyed had missed or delayed a medical appointment because they were anxious about contracting the virus in hospital, and over half reported being anxious or lonely. Audet's (2020) study in Belgium found that the pandemic had increased women's anxieties, especially about hospitals and medical services. Pregnant women perceived hospitals as COVID-19 hotspots. If they had to go into hospital, then they felt there was an 'atmosphere of war' as the PPE worn by staff prevented any intimacy. Many services were receiving phone calls from pregnant women requesting home births, which were denied 'on the basis that home birth cannot be motivated by fear' (Audet, 2020).

Ashworth (2020) commented that 'a worrying and persistent theme has been the removal of a variety of service options, which were justified as being for the safety of women', but in reality were to protect staff. Audet (2020) noted that hospitals in Belgium adopted protocols to minimise infections, but since each hospital adopted its own measures, it created 'a climate of distrust and confusion'. In some cases, women were offered caesarean sections that were not medically indicated, which could result in 'obstetric violence'. Rosamund Urwin, who reflected on her own and other mothers' experiences of being pregnant and giving birth during the pandemic, commented: 'Pregnant women have been one of the forgotten groups in the pandemic' (2021, p. 24).

Comment

Public health experts tend to focus on dangers of specific illnesses. Foregrounding such risk can and does provide ways of protecting individuals, but it fails to recognise that in everyday life individuals do not face and have

Table 3.3: Implications of the precautionary principle

1. Categorisation as high risk
a. Heyman et al have observed (2010, p. 46) those placed in a high-risk category are treated as if they are in imminent danger; however, the actual absolute risk of such a negative outcome may be low
b. Being placed in the high-risk category can have negative impacts on those categorised in this way, by, for example, changing their self-perceptions and perceptions of others, resulting in restrictions of activities and unnecessary treatments
c. Experts, especially when their remit centres on a specific risk such as COVID-19 infection, will foreground this risk
2. Single versus multiple risks
a. Experts foregrounding one risk, such as the risk of COVID-19 infection, play down other risks that may be equally harmful and/or be more likely
b. In their everyday lives, individuals such as pregnant women have to identify and manage a range of risks
c. A high-risk categorisation may impede a pregnant woman's agency by denying her access and support to manage non-COVID-19 risks

to deal with a single risk but have to balance multiple risks. By increasing the social isolation of pregnant women (and reducing their access to health services and pre-natal care), policy makers (inadvertently) contributed to their increased anxiety and depression, and reduced their capacity to manage the different risks they faced (see Table 3.3).

Case Study 3: Deciding on priorities for the COVID-19 vaccine

The development and approval of COVID-19 vaccines in late 2020 provided a way of controlling and bringing the pandemic to an end. Policy makers had to decide who to prioritise for the vaccinations. Different countries adopted rather different processes, chose different priorities and highlighted different risks.

Mechanisms for choosing

Countries differed in the mechanisms they used to decide on priorities. Such differences reflected their political and policy-making structures. For example, in the Russian Federation there was no public or scientific debate about priorities: the decision was made by the political leadership and announced in a decree issued by the president, Vladimir Putin (Litvinova, 2020). In China, decision making is centralised and controlled by the Communist Party, so priorities were established by an expert committee that formed part of the State Council (The Central People's Government of the People's Republic of China, 2020).

In high-income democratic countries, the key input to prioritisation came ostensibly from experts and an element of transparency was aimed for. In

France, planning for vaccination started in July 2020 with the publication of a scientific advisory committee report (CARE, 2020). The committee reviewed the science, making recommendations to central government about vaccination priorities. The government also decided to consult the public in order to assess public preferences. This was time consuming, but enabled the government to 'understand what people value' (Roope et al, 2020).

In Germany, the federal government recognised that priorities should not be based solely on medical/epidemiological issues but should also be informed by ethical and legal considerations (The Joint Working Party, 2020). The Federal Ministry of Health invited a working party, made up of members of the Standing Committee on Vaccination, experts from the National Academy of Sciences Leopoldina and from the German Ethics Council, to establish a framework for fair prioritisation (The Joint Working Party, 2020). The working party developed a detailed vaccination programme based on this framework.

In the US and UK, the government effectively delegated the decision to medical/epidemiological experts. In the US, the CDC made decisions on vaccination programmes based on the recommendations of the Advisory Committee on Immunization Practices (ACIP). The 15 voting experts of ACIP were appointed by Federal Department of Health and Human Services based on applications and nominations. While there were 14 voting members who had expertise in health issues such as vaccinology, public health and infectious diseases, and one was a consumer representative, there were also 30 non-voting members representing various health professions. The committee excluded individuals with connections to the pharmaceutical industry. It met at least three times a year, with its meetings open to the public and available as online webcasts. Prior to each voting session, there was time for oral public comment as well as the opportunity for written submissions (CDC, 2021c).

In the UK, there was a centralised system of decision making and no public consultation. The Joint Committee on Vaccination and Immunisation (JCVI), which was made up of scientists with specialist knowledge about the development of vaccines and their distribution (JCVI, 2020b), recommended priorities for vaccination. Most of the members (14 out of 16) were experts in respiratory diseases, virology or vaccine development.

Vaccination priorities: making choices between risks and values

In countries in which the main risk of the pandemic was seen as economic disruption, priority was given to vaccinating younger and economically more active individuals. For example, in the Russian Federation, workers, especially those most exposed to the virus through their work in health, social care and education, were given top priority. Older people were excluded from the programme: no one over 60 was to receive the vaccine

(Soldatkin, 2020). Similarly in Indonesia, the government decided to give priority to vaccination of people aged 18–59 to protect the workforce and boost the economy. A spokesman for the Ministry of Health noted that the younger age group 'plays an important role in economic activities that support families...' and that vaccinating them could 'break the chain of transmission in the family cluster', reducing infection rates (Ekawati, 2021).

France, on the other hand, developed a mixed strategy for vaccination, protecting those at risk – whether workers whose jobs made them vulnerable or those whose age, health or living conditions exposed them to greater risk. In July 2020, the scientific advisory committee (CARE, 2020) reviewed the evidence and identified a top tier of priorities

- Groups at risk because of their work (c 6.8 million), of whom 1.8 million were the highest priority. This highest priority group included front-line health-care staff and those in contact with vulnerable populations.
- Groups at risk because of their age or state of health (c 23 million). Of these, nearly 13.5 million were 65 or over, 4 million were under 65 but had underlying health problems and 10 million were obese.
- Individuals living in situations of high vulnerability (c 250,000). These included those living in hostels or squats.

Following government consultation, the final guidelines included in the top priority group those working in high-risk jobs, including health workers, shop workers, school staff, transport staff such as taxi drivers, hospitality workers and abattoir staff (Roope et al, 2020).

In China, the State Council subcommittee also proposed a mixed strategy that prioritised two high-risk groups for vaccination; key workers and vulnerable individuals who were at risk of severe illness if infected (The Central People's Government of the People's Republic of China, 2020). The key worker group included front-line medical and infection control workers, port and border workers, workers providing key services in cities and those who had to travel to areas with high infection rates. The at-risk group included the elderly, children, pregnant women and people with underlying diseases.

In Germany, valuing and protecting the most vulnerable was the priority. The Joint Working Party started with an ethical framework for its prioritisation that identified four key ethical and legal issues. From these, it identified four guiding goals for the vaccination programme:

- Prevention of severe cases of COVID-19 that result in hospitalisation and deaths.
- Protection of persons with an especially high work-related risk of exposure to the virus.

- Prevention of transmission and protection in environments with a high proportion of vulnerable individuals and in those with a high outbreak potential.
- Maintenance of essential state functions and public life. (The Joint Committee, 2020, p. 3)

The working party argued that in view of the urgency of the situation, goal 1 was the main one, so the first priority should be given to individuals who were at risk of serious or fatal illness because of their age or underlying illness, especially if they lived in settings such as nursing homes where they had close contact with other vulnerable individuals (The Joint Working Party, 2020, p. 3).

The working party noted that alongside the urgency of the situation, there was also a need to consider social solidarity. Therefore, individuals who through their work were at risk or who were a risk to others if they transmitted the virus should be the second priority. This group included health service employees and those working in facilities for the elderly (The Joint Working Party, 2020, p. 3). The working party also noted that individuals who performed key services that were essential to state and public life should be protected by vaccines. These included employees of local health authorities, police and security agencies, fire brigades, teachers and educators (The Joint Committee, 2020, p. 3).

In the UK, the JCVI identified priorities for vaccination in December 2020 (JCVI, 2020a, p. 8). The committee began by considering three possible goals for a vaccination programme:

- Distributing vaccines as quickly as possible using procedures established for seasonal flu vaccination.
- Achieving social justice by prioritising communities experiencing social deprivation and relatively high levels of infection and deaths.
- Reducing the transmission of the virus.

Given the urgency of the situation, the JCVI chose the first goal, recommending priority be given to the most vulnerable and those who care for them. The committee recommended that the vaccination programme should focus on the over 50s, starting with residents in care homes for older adults and their carers, followed by individuals over 80 years old and front-line health and social care workers, then individuals over 75 years followed by individuals aged 70 and over and those who were extremely clinically vulnerable (JCVI, 2020a, p. 8). The JCVI explicitly excluded pregnant women from the vaccination programme, observing that 'Given the lack of evidence, JCVI favours a precautionary approach and does not currently advise COVID-19 vaccination in pregnancy' (JCVI, 2020a, p. 5).

In making its decision, the JCVI identified three ethical principles that should inform the priorities:

- maximisation of benefit and reduction of harm;
- promotion of transparency and fairness;
- mitigation of health inequalities. (JCVI, 2020a, pp 17–18)

The JCVI adopted a utilitarian approach that maximised the net benefit to society by minimising harm, especially serious illness, hospitalisations and death. The experts advising the JCVI argued that

> From an ethical perspective, prioritisation should maximise benefit and reduce harm. Scientific evidence … allows us to focus on populations that are at highest risk of infection, hospitalisation, and death from COVID-19. It is important that these population groups are the first to receive the vaccine, as they are the most likely to benefit from them. (JCVI, 2020a, p. 17)

The JCVI justified its priority list in pragmatic terms, noting that: 'Simple age-based programmes are usually easier to deliver and therefore achieve higher uptake including in the highest risk groups' (JCVI, 2020a, p. 16).

There has been little public discussion of the priorities in the UK. One of the few critical commentaries came from Alexis Paton, an academic with an interest in medical ethics. Paton argued that priority should be given to the most vulnerable in society, but that vulnerability should not be judged just in terms of age and underlying illness; rather, it should include social factors such as deprivation. She noted that such choices reflected social values and 'how we value or do not value, certain members of [society]' (Paton, 2020, p. 9).

The priorities that different governments adopted for COVID-19 vaccination reflected their preferred outcomes and the values on which those outcomes were based. Governments that prioritised vaccinating younger and economically active cohorts were willing to tolerate serious illness and death among more vulnerable groups. In contrast, those that prioritised high-risk groups accepted the continued disruption of the lives of younger people who worked or were in education to protect the lives of those who were more vulnerable if infected.

Comment

Quantifying risk involves assessing the probability of different outcomes and judging the relative values of these outcomes. During the pandemic, policy makers were comfortable with the technicalities of risk, acknowledging the probability of infection and death. They were far less comfortable acknowledging the difficult choices that had to be made, and how these involved valuing and distributing benefits and illness between different social groups. In the UK, the CMO, Chris Whitty, observed that deaths during pandemics were inevitable, but deciding what level was tolerable should not be a decision for experts: 'that's a political decision. That's a societal decision' (Rev, 2021).

However, as I have argued, in high-income countries policy makers are unwilling to explicitly identify and own the value systems that underpin their decisions; indeed, the use of risk as an apparently technical neutral concept effectively masks and conceals these value decisions. In the UK, the JCVI (2020b) is an advisory body, so ministers can choose whether or not they accept its advice. During the pandemic, Conservative ministers were happy to accept advice that prioritised their core supporters, older, male and White voters. There was no effective challenge to these decisions from the opposition parties, which draw their core support from younger people, women and ethnic minority groups, those effectively excluded from the priority list.

4

Communicating risk: public health messaging

Risk: the challenge of communication

Public health campaigns are designed to make the public aware of specific risks and to change collective behaviour in order to minimise those risks. These campaigns often use emotions, such as anxiety, fear and guilt, to foreground and attract public attention to the specific risk and the associated collective behavioural change needed to mitigate it. This approach has underpinned campaigns such as the UK's regular 'don't drink and drive' campaigns (The Telegraph, 2020) and was evident in the 1980s with the 'don't die of ignorance' HIV/AIDS campaign (Burgess, 2017). In Australia in July 2021, the federal government was criticised for using scare tactics when it released a COVID-19 awareness advert that showed a young women in a hospital bed fighting for breath (Wahliquist, 2021).

Achieving the right balance

Public messaging needs to achieve a balance between creating enough anxiety to engender desired changes in behaviour, but not so much that there are adverse reactions. Quigley (2005) examines the ways in which governments in the US and UK sought to manage one major risk, the so-called Millennium Bug: the danger that at midnight on 1 January 2000 computer systems would crash, as many used a two-digit system that would not be able to differentiate 2000 from 1900. Both governments engaged in public awareness campaigns, and these were so successful that by the end of 1998, the US government was seeking to reduce public anxiety and avoid panic reactions such as hoarding (Quigley, 2005, p. 288).

To communicate effectively, policy makers and health promoters need to convert their information about risks and how to mitigate them into messages that can be understood and acted on by their target audiences. The effectiveness of such messaging depends on how they are structured (the source) and the ways in which they are received and used by target audiences (the reception). Jetten and colleagues (2020) have considered the ways in which messages should be delivered. They argue that the purpose of risk communication should not be to punish or force individuals to comply with government diktats; rather, 'The role of governments should

Table 4.1: Factors that contribute to the successful communication of risk messages

The messages and messengers	Hearing and acting on messages
openness and honesty of the source	the extent to which the source of the information is trusted
source shows respect for the public	the relevance of the information for everyday life and decision making
message ensures equity, so everyone is treated the same	the relation to other perceived risks
message is consistent	the fit with previous knowledge and experience
message makes clear that 'we are all in it together'	the difficulty and importance of the choices and decisions

Source: Alaszewski and Horlick-Jones (2003) and Reicher in Social Science Space (2020)

be to support and enlist this public resilience' (Jetten et al, 2020, p. 14). Reicher (2020) has identified five elements that contribute to a successful risk communication strategy (see Table 4.1). Alaszewski and Horlick-Jones (2003) have reflected on how messages are received. They argue that the response of target audiences depends on their trust in the source of message, the clarity of the message and its relevance to their lives (see Table 4.1).

First- and second-order observers

Drawing on the work of Luhmann (1993), Kiisel and Vihalemm (2014) developed a framework to examine how and why risk messages that warn of dangers are accepted or rejected. Luhmann argues that an individual response to information depends on whether they are first-order or second-order observers. First-order observers directly observe an event and can treat what they observe as facts about the real world. In terms of risk, first-order observers can ask 'How dangerous is this situation and what should I do about it?' Second-order observers do not directly observe events but have to rely on the observations of others. They may reflect on the role of first order observers and whether they are selecting or withholding facts, asking, 'How accurate is their representation of the situation and can I trust their representation?' Thus for Luhmann (1993, pp 1–31), risk-taking is intertwined with communication: second-order observers have to decide which messenger and messages to trust and accept and which to distrust and reject. As Kiisel and Vihalemm (2014) note, such decisions are not made in a vacuum: individuals build up trust or distrust in sources of risk messages. 'In modern societies, the guiding rationale for individuals in their responses to warning messages is often their previous experience: many risks that at are initially ignored are reassessed later and, *vice versa*, many risks are seen, in retrospect, as overstated' (Kiisel and Vihalemm, 2014, p. 279). They go on to say that individuals tend to place more trust in those they perceive to be neutral or independent, such as researchers and civic movements, and less in those who they perceive to have a vested interest, such as government officials and politicians. Kiisel and Vihalemm (2014, p. 281) argue that the response of individuals to warning messages is shaped by two key elements: the extent to which an individual's personal experience fits in with observations contained in the warning message and the degree to which individuals accept that the proposed response to the danger has been shown to work.

Kiisel and Vihalemm (2014) examined the ways in which individuals in focus groups in Estonia responded to warning about three potential dangers: storms, a radiation leak from a nuclear power station and possible chemical pollution. They found that responses to warnings were shaped by whether the warnings conformed to first-order observations. Participants accepted the storm and the danger it represented as a 'given' because 'a storm is a storm' (Kiisel and Vihalemm, 2014, p. 284). In contrast, participants had no direct experience of technological accidents such as a radiation leak, and struggled to name the uncertainty it represented. Their reaction was one of increased anxiety about the danger rather than a search for more information. When participants felt that message and proposed protective action fitted with their experience then they were happy to follow guidance; for example, 'they "would stay at home" (in the case of the storm warning)' (Kiisel and Vihalemm, 2014, p. 285). However, when they were uncertain about or distrusted the source of the information and the proposed course of action, they looked to their own more familiar and trusted sources of information. This was particularly the case for technological accidents: some 'participants treated the institutions that issued the warnings as trustworthy [but] were aware of their potential fallibility' (Kiisel and Vihalemm, 2014, p. 287).

Individuals in most countries are familiar with infectious diseases and illnesses such as the common cold and flu. However, in early 2020, COVID-19 represented a distinctive and novel danger, a pandemic disease, one that infected large sections of the population at the same time and required large-scale coordinated action to protect the population from the worst consequences. In the reminder of this chapter, I consider the ways in which national governments sought to communicate the danger and recommended protections, and the effectiveness of their communications.

Communicating the public health message during the pandemic

Developing and communicating a consistent risk message

The challenge of communicating the risks of COVID-19 was affected by the ways in which it was initially framed. In those countries in which it was initially framed as a SARS or Ebola-like disease, there was no need to change the public health message. From the start, the new virus was presented as a major danger and one that required significant changes in behaviour.

Taiwan had a rapid response to COVID-19 that included consistent risk messaging. Following the initial identification of COVID-19, the government set up the Central Epidemic Command Centre within the National Health Command Centre to coordinate the collection and dissemination of information about COVID-19. The aim was to keep everyone in the country well informed, enabling a community-wide response to the virus. The messaging from the government explained travel restrictions and outlined social distancing rules and personal hygiene recommendations such as the universal use of face masks (Chen, 2020). The authorities backed up these broad messages with specific information designed to help residents follow the guidelines. For example, to help citizens access supplies of face masks, the Taiwanese government released real-time information on mask stocks so suppliers could use mobile phone map apps to provide up-to-date information about the make and availability of masks and safe pick-up locations (Hung, 2020).

As I note in Chapter 2, Japan, although it was on the western Pacific Rim, did not initially frame the new virus as SARS-like but downplayed its dangerousness. In March 2020, there was no evidence of COVID-19 clusters in Japan, but the government began to warn the population of the danger and advised changing behaviours to reduce the risk of spread. On 26 March, the Government Expert Group on COVID-19 indicated that 'there was a "high probability of the expansion of infections," in light of the increase in infection cases entering from overseas' (Government of Japan, 2020, p. 1). This expert group sponsored a unique 'Japan model' that focused on 'modifying the behaviour of citizens and early detecting and responding to clusters' (Government of Japan, 2020, p. 5). This was based on engaging citizens and encouraging them to change their behaviour to avoid infection by providing clear information on the places and behaviours to avoid:

> The locations where mass infections were confirmed so far are places where the following three conditions were met simultaneously: (1) closed space with poor ventilation, (2) crowded with many people and (3) conversations and vocalization in close proximity (within arm's reach of one another). It is believed that more people were infected in such places. Therefore, we ask that you predict locations and settings where these three conditions could occur simultaneously and avoid them. We do not have enough scientific evidence yet on how significantly such actions can reduce the risk of spreading infection. However, since places with poor ventilation and crowded places are increasing infections, we ask that you take precautions even before scientific evidence for clear standards is found.(Government of Japan, 2020, p. 2)

This low-key approach to COVID-19 and the plea for cooperation from the Japanese people was also evident in a speech made by Prime Minister Shinzo Abe on 2 March. He said: 'We are aware we are causing trouble for the Japanese people [by asking for their cooperation in social distancing] but we also humbly ask cooperation from each and every person' (McGrath, 2020).

While the relatively low-key response of Shinzo Abe and the Japanese government to COVID-19 has been criticised in Japan (McGrath, 2020), the country was relatively successful in controlling infection and death rates. 18 months into the pandemic and following the Olympic Games in 2021, Japan remained in the intermediate group of countries in terms of infections (nearly 1.7 million confirmed cases) and deaths (17,475 – 13.84 per 100,000 compared with the UK's 7.5 million cases and 136,465 deaths – 204.18 per 100,000) (Johns Hopkins University of Medicine, 2021). The initial success of Japan in containing the virus seemed to relate to the receptiveness of the Japanese to social distancing messages. Elements of traditional Japanese culture were well suited to social distancing. For example, the Japanese were aware of and sought to protect the symbolic boundaries of both the household and the body. It is conventional in Japan to protect the household by removing outside shoes when crossing the threshold. Indeed, inviting visitors into the house is unusual. Similarly, attention is paid to protecting the entry to the body, the mouth, and wearing masks is normal and socially acceptable (Alaszewska and Alaszewski, 2015).

Mixed messages: public health messaging in the UK and US

In countries that initially framed COVID-19 as flu-like, such as the UK and US, there were major shifts in messaging, especially in the early stages of the pandemic when it became evident that there was community transmission and that hospital admissions and deaths were rising rapidly. In some countries, such as the US, the messaging was undermined by tensions between populist politicians and public health experts.

Messaging in the UK

In early March, there was a debate in the UK government about COVID-19 risk and how best to manage it, and some of the discussion was communicated with the public. For example, in a press conference on 10 March, Prime Minister Boris Johnson reflected on the options available to respond to the spread of the virus. He discussed the possibility of adopting 'draconian measures' such as stopping public gatherings, cancelling public events and closing schools, but also reflected on the possibility of allowing the virus to spread and that perhaps 'you could take it on the chin, take it all in one go and allow the disease, as it were, to move through the population, without taking as many draconian measures. I think we need to strike a balance … [between measures to control the virus and allowing it to spread]' (Full Fact, 2020).

The message in early March was unclear and to some extent muddled. It seemed to be that while the virus was a danger especially to vulnerable people, the majority of the population should as far as possible carry on as normal, making their own assessments of the risks. This mixed messaging could be seen in specific areas such as hand hygiene. On 3 March, behavioural experts on the Independent Scientific Pandemic Insights Group on Behaviours (SPI-B) stated 'that government should advise against greetings such as shaking hands and hugging, given existing evidence about the importance of hand hygiene' (Woodward, 2020b). On 3 March, the prime minister said: 'I was at a hospital the other night where I think there were actually a few coronavirus patients and I shook hands with everybody' (Woodward, 2020b). He continued shaking hands in public until 9 March (Woodward, 2020b).

In late March 2020, the UK government shifted from a wait and see approach, with all options open, to lockdown, necessitating a major shift in messaging. Personal behaviour was no longer to be based on personal risk assessments but on a state-mandated requirement to minimise social contact. In his statement on 17 March announcing lockdown, the prime minister asked the public to trust his judgement that it was the right moment to change policy:

> And if you ask, 'Well, why are we doing this now? Why now? Why not earlier or later? Why bring in this very draconian measure,' the answer is that we are asking people to do something that is difficult and disruptive of their lives. And the right moment, as we've always said, is to do it when it is most effective, when we think it can make the biggest difference to slowing the spread of the disease, reducing the number of victims, reducing the number of fatalities. (Rev, 2020a)

The effectiveness of this 'trust-me' message depends on the public perception of the trustworthiness of the messenger. To reinforce trustworthiness, Boris Johnson's words were endorsed by two experts, the CSA, Sir Patrick Vallance, and CMO, Chris Whitty. Patrick Vallance provided the scientific justification for the measures, stating that it was based on a rational plan and advice from the expert advisory committee, SAGE:

> This is a very fast-moving situation. The latest numbers that we reviewed at SAGE suggest that we're entering a fast-growth period or on the cusp of doing so, and London is ahead of other parts of the country. We at the outset laid out a plan and advised that we would implement it, the measures, at the right stage and in the right

combination, the right combination to ensure that we get the biggest impact. Unfortunately, that time is now for many of these measures. … The measures have two objectives. One is to delay the transmission of this virus across the community, and the second is to keep people safe. (Rev, 2020a)

While there was public mistrust of politicians in general, and Boris Johnson in particular thanks to his divisive populist politics, there appears to have been more trust in medical and scientific experts such as Chris Whitty and Patrick Vallance. As in the US, trust in health experts was a more significant factor in influencing the uptake of protective actions than trust in political leadership in influencing the uptake of protective actions, 58 per cent of a sample of US citizens trusted health experts compared with 18 per cent who trusted the White House leadership. Those who trusted health experts were more likely to take actions to protect themselves and others from the virus (Ahluwalia et al, 2021). The first lockdown in the UK was accepted with little dissent. The public generally accepted the warning that SARS-CoV-2 was a major threat and accepted social distancing advice as there appeared to be no alternative.

The messaging in March 2020 was not linked to a clear decision framework that provided simple and easy-to-grasp signals. Instead, policy makers referred to various indicators such as R_0 (rate of transmission), infection rates, hospital and ICU admissions and death rates. These indicators were used to justify the initial lockdown at the end of March and its easing in June.

When a second set of restrictions became necessary in late summer in specific parts of the UK, there were communication problems. In late July, the prime minister announced increased social distancing measures in the north of England based on data indicating increased levels of infection. This evidence was disputed; for example, Carl Heneghan suggested the rise was a product of skewed data and that 'the northern lockdown was a rash decision' (Knapton, 2020). To simplify the messaging in England, policy makers used a three-tier alert system, with limited restrictions for those living in Tier 1 and severe restrictions for those living in Tier 3. This system failed to reduce infection levels, resulting in a second England-wide lockdown in November 2020 followed by a new four-tier system of restrictions. This in turn failed to control the virus, leading to a third national lockdown in January 2021 (Rev, 2021).

The difficulties of communicating risk and ensuring compliance with safety measures was increased by the perception that policy makers were asking citizens to obey rules that they themselves ignored with impunity. The most commented-on case occurred in May 2020 when the prime minister's special advisor, Dominic Cummings, flouted lockdown measures by making a 300-mile trip to Durham, including a day trip to a local town, Barnard Castle (Rutter, 2020, pp 7–8).

Mixed messaging in the US

In the US, the relationship between the president and his scientific advisers was tense and fractious. During the early stages of the pandemic, the president did accept some expert advice. For example, Woodward documents (2020a, pp 280–6) the ways in which the key policy shift from wait and see to lockdown was shaped by discussions between experts, the president and his inner circle. In public, the president claimed credit for the decision. At a meeting of the Coronavirus Task Force on 17 March 2020, Donald Trump claimed that 'I've always known this is a – this is real – this is a pandemic. I've felt this is a pandemic long before it was called a pandemic' (Woodward, 2020a, pp 285–6).

As the pandemic developed in early summer 2020, tensions between the president and his expert advisers became more evident. There were differences over: treatment regimes, with the president advocating unproven treatments such as hydrochloroquine, public health messaging about wearing face masks, and the ending of the first lockdown. The Trump team marginalised public health experts such as Anthony Fauci, appointing a press secretary who limited Fauci's television appearances. Fauci did occasionally contradict Trump in public, but commented that if the president made incorrect statements in public, 'I can't jump in front of the microphone and push him down' (Woodward, 2020a, p. 353).

The relationship between Donald Trump and scientists and public health experts deteriorated to such an extent that it became open conflict. *Scientific American*, which promotes non-partisan science, published an editorial endorsing Joe Biden in October 2020:

> The evidence and the science show that Donald Trump has badly damaged the U.S. and its people – because he rejects evidence and science. The most devastating example is his dishonest and inept response to the COVID-19 pandemic, which cost more than 190,000 Americans their lives by the middle of September. (*Scientific American*, 2020)

Despite this, Donald Trump retained a strong core of supporters, who trusted him and refused to accept that COVID-19 was a life threatening illness; and while he lost the presidential election in November 2020, it was not by a wide margin. As I have already noted, 18 per cent of respondents in a sample of US citizens indicated that they trusted the White House leadership (Ahluwalia et al, 2021). I return to this issue in Chapter 8 where I consider why so many people mistrusted experts during the COVID-19 pandemic and examines conspiracy theories and contested risk during the pandemic.

Case Study 4: Engendering and maintaining trust through effective risk communication in New Zealand

Initial communication of the risk of COVID-19

In New Zealand, the initial public health message was cautious. On 28 January 2020, the government issued the first public assessment of risk, noting that 'while the risk of spread to New Zealand is low, the current outbreak in China of novel coronavirus is capable of being transmitted between human beings and poses a potentially serious risk to public health' (New Zealand Cabinet Office, 2020).

However, to minimise the risk of COVID-19 spreading to New Zealand, the government decided to 'address the public health risk of transmission of the novel coronavirus in New Zealand'. It categorised 'the novel coronavirus capable of causing severe respiratory illness' as a notifiable disease that could be managed using existing powers to control infectious diseases (New Zealand Cabinet Office, 2020).

Using a risk framework to communicate risk

When it became clear in March that the virus had reached New Zealand, the government developed a system of alert levels to communicate the overall risk to the public, together with the actions the government wanted individuals and organisations to take to mitigate the risks of COVID-19 (Wilson, 2020) (see Table 4.2). The system provided:

- A rationale for decisions made in the present: The framework was introduced on Saturday 21 March 2020, at the time that New Zealand was moving into lockdown. On Monday 23 March, Jacinda Ardern, the prime minister, announced national lockdown, and used the risk framework as the justification for her decision (Ardern, 2020a).
- A way of mapping and providing hope for the future: As New Zealand moved into lockdown, there was a clear way out. In her speech announcing the lockdown, Ardern provided a timeframe for moving from Level 4 lockdown:

   If we flush out the cases we already have and see transmission slow, we will potentially be able to move areas out of Level 4 over time. ... If we after those 4 weeks we have been successful [in stopping community transmission], we hope we will be able to ease up on restrictions. If we haven't, we'll find ourselves living with them for longer. (Ardern, 2020a)

- A way of reflecting on the past: Policy makers could use the alert system to reflect on the success of actions and warnings. On 8 June, Ardern reflected on the success of the lockdown:

Table 4.2: New Zealand alert system

	Alert Level 1 Prepare	Alert Level 2 Reduce	Alert Level 3 Restrict	Alert Level 4 Lockdown
Risk assessment	COVID-19 is uncontrolled overseas	The disease is contained, but the risk of community transmission remains	High risk, the disease is not contained	Likely that the disease is not contained
	Sporadic imported cases	Limited community transmission could be occurring	Multiple cases of community transmission occurring	Sustained and intensive community transmission is occurring
	Isolated local transmission could be occurring in New Zealand	Active clusters in more than one region	Multiple active clusters in multiple regions.	Widespread outbreaks
Individual and collective actions	Border entry measures to minimise risk of importing COVID-19 cases	People can connect with friends and family, and socialise in groups of up to 100	People instructed to stay at home in their bubble other than for essential personal movement, work school or recreation	People instructed to stay at home in their bubble other than for essential personal movement
	Intensive testing for COVID-19	Keep physical distancing of 2 metres from people. Keep 1 metre physical distancing in workplaces	Physical distancing of 2 metres outside home, or 1 metre in controlled environments	Safe recreational activity is allowed in local area
	Rapid contact tracing of any positive case	No more than 100 people at gatherings	Legally, people must stay within their immediate household bubble, but can expand this to connect with close family/caregivers, or to support isolated people	Travel is severely limited

Table 4.2: New Zealand alert system (continued)

	Alert Level 1 Prepare	Alert Level 2 Reduce	Alert Level 3 Restrict	Alert Level 4 Lockdown
	Self-isolation and quarantine required	Businesses can open to the public if following public health guidance	Schools, years 1 to 10, and early childhood education centres can safely open, but will have limited capacity	All gatherings cancelled and all public venues closed
	Schools and workplaces open	Hospitality businesses must keep groups of customers separated, seated and served by a single person	People must work from home unless that is not possible	Businesses closed except for essential services. For example, supermarkets, pharmacies, clinics, petrol stations and lifeline utilities
	No restrictions on personal movement, but people are encouraged to maintain a record of where they have been	Sport and recreation activities are allowed, subject to conditions on gatherings	Businesses cannot offer services that involve close personal contact, unless it is a supermarket, pharmacy, petrol station, or it is an emergency or critical situation	Educational facilities closed
	No restrictions on gatherings, but organisers encouraged to maintain records to enable contact tracing	Public venues can open if they comply with public health measures	Other businesses can open premises, but cannot physically interact with customers. Low-risk local recreation activities are allowed	Rationing of supplies and requisitioning of facilities possible
	Stay home if you're sick, report flu-like symptoms	Event facilities, including cinemas, stadiums, concert venues and casinos, can have more than 100 people at a time	Low-risk local recreation activities are allowed	Reprioritisation of health-care services

Note: Some of the prescribed actions have been omitted

Source: New Zealand Government (2020)

A lot has happened since we were first at Alert Level 2 in late March, prior to entering Alert Level 4. We took strong early action against the spread of COVID-19, closing the borders to passengers, moving up Alert Levels, and imposing a lock down when we had reported only a small number of cases. We saw high compliance with the rules by New Zealanders and high levels of public support for our actions despite their social, economic and fiscal costs. And our collective efforts have paid off. For now, we can have high confidence that we have eliminated COVID-19 within New Zealand, i.e. that there are no more infected people in our population. (Ardern, 2020b)

- A clear rationale for differential responses to the virus in different parts of the country: In August 2020, the government responded to a cluster of cases in the capital, Auckland, by retaining a higher alert level in the area (Ward, 2020).

The alert framework provided an effective base for public health messaging and formed the basis of simple slogans: 'Stay home, stay safe, and be kind' and 'United against COVID-19'. Such messaging linked risk mitigation (stay safe) to reinforcing behaviours designed to protect (stay home) and support the community (be kind) (Goodman, 2020). In her speech announcing the lockdown, Jacinda Ardern stressed the collective benefits of individual behavioural change. By using the pronoun 'we' rather than 'you', she represented lockdown as a joint and collective enterprise (Ardern, 2020a).

In appealing to the altruism of the New Zealand population and asking them to make collective sacrifices for the common good, Ardern and her government were asking for the population's trust: trust in government and trust in fellow citizens. There were to be no exceptions: those connected with the government had to follow the same rules as the rest of the population. In New Zealand, this aspect of trust was undermined by the behaviour of the health minister, who twice breached the lockdown rules. Initially, he apologised, was demoted and publicly criticised by Ardern (Roy, 2020). Following continued public criticism, he resigned in July 2020 (BBC, 2020a).

Risk implications

New Zealand adopted a zero-COVID-19 policy, and public health messaging contributed to the success of that policy. In the first 18 months of the pandemic, New Zealand had 4,184 confirmed cases of COVID-19 and 27 COVID-19 related deaths, a rate of 0.55 per 100,000 (Johns Hopkins University of Medicine, 2021). In the early stages of the pandemic, the government clearly warned the population of the dangers. It then developed and used a risk framework to justify the introduction of social distancing measures and then to relax them. The government was able to present its strategy as fair, just and inclusive through its 'be kind' message and by punishing ministers who breached the guidelines. In retrospect, Jacinda Ardern may regret that she did not sack her health minister earlier. This would have sent a clearer message that 'we are all in this together'.

Case Study 5: Public health messaging about COVID-19 vaccines and vaccine hesitancy

The messages

It is relatively straightforward to identify and analyse public health messages. It is, however, more difficult to examine how and why individuals and social groups chose to respond to such messages in a variety of ways. The messaging around COVID-19 vaccines provides an opportunity to examine such responses. The public health messaging around vaccines was clear. The message was that the vaccines were safe, they had major personal benefits reducing the risk of serious illness and death, and had important collective benefits, including reducing the risk of transmission. On its website, the CDC outlined the benefits of getting a COVID-19 vaccine:

COVID-19 vaccines are safe
- While COVID-19 vaccines were developed rapidly, all steps have been taken to ensure their safety and effectiveness.
- COVID-19 vaccines were developed using science that has been around for decades.
- COVID-19 vaccines are not experimental. They went through all the required stages of clinical trials. Extensive testing and monitoring have shown that these vaccines are safe and effective.
- COVID-19 vaccines have received and continue to undergo the most intensive safety monitoring in U.S. history.

COVID-19 vaccines are effective
- COVID-19 vaccines are effective. They can keep you from getting and spreading the virus that causes COVID-19.
- COVID-19 vaccines also help keep you from getting seriously ill even if you do get COVID-19.
- Getting vaccinated yourself may also protect people around you, particularly people at increased risk for severe illness from COVID-19
- After you are fully vaccinated for COVID-19, you can resume many activities that you did before the pandemic. (CDC, 2021d)

Disregarding public health messaging; a rational choice?

It is tempting to see the disregarding of public health messaging as ignorance (not hearing the messages) or irrationality (failing to understand the significance of the warnings). In response to evidence that one-third of the US military had declined COVID-19 vaccination, Anthony Fauci observed that these individuals were 'inadvertently being part of the problem'. He observed that military personnel has a civic duty to accept the vaccine: 'Because by getting infected, even though you may not know it, you may be inadvertently transmitting the infection to someone else, even though you have no symptoms ... in reality, like it or not, you're propagating this outbreak' (Hart, 2021).

The response of experts to vaccine hesitancy was measured. However, in the social media debate on vaccination, there were more critical comments. For example, Piers Morgan, an outspoken media commentator, tweeted: 'People have the right to not get vaccinated against covid. Just as I have the right to think they're selfish, deluded ignorant morons who will keep this pandemic going much longer than it should. #GetJabbed' (Morgan, 2021).

Individuals choosing not to vaccinate have often done so in full knowledge of the expert advice. In an article on employment law and vaccination, an employment lawyer reflected on his conversation with a colleague whom he regarded as a rational and intelligent person whose opinions he had always held in high regard:

> The other day one of my closest lawyer friends outed herself to me as a Covid vaccination sceptic. She dropped this casually into a conversation, mentioning in passing that she hadn't had the vaccine. Taken aback, I asked her if she had missed her appointment. 'No,' she said. 'I just don't believe in it. It's not been properly tested. I don't trust our politicians. And frankly, I don't think it's the best way of stopping Covid. (Alaszewski, 2021b)

As Mary Douglas observed, decisions to disregard warnings and to take risks that can result in serious harm, even death, are cultural choices that reflect an individual's identity as a risk taker and their relationship to wider social networks they are a part of. She reflected on such choices in the context of the HIV/AIDS pandemic when individuals, especially gay men, were warned about unprotected sex. Drawing on research on HIV/AIDS in France, Douglas and Calvez (1990) observed that the gay community formed an excluded community whose members rejected the values of the dominant society and the warnings grounded in these values:

As to being a population at risk, the definition meets an ethos that glorifies risk. Many in such a community would deride the cult of safety. Death comes to all in the end. Who would want to live a safe life if that means no passion, no ecstasy, no abandon. The idea of a high risk life style is an accepted norm. (Douglas and Calvez, 1990, p. 461)

Thus, while decisions about vaccines are taken by individuals, as Douglas and Calvez observed, individuals belong to social groups, and their decisions will be influenced by these groups.

Policy makers and public health experts have expressed concern about vaccine hesitancy and the way it undermines the collective response to the pandemic, the achievement of herd immunity. The Organisation for Economic Co-operation and Development (OECD) noted the scientific consensus that 'the most effective way to defeat the COVID-19 pandemic is through the mass vaccination of populations around the world' (OECD, 2021). The OECD identified significant vaccine hesitancy in the high-income countries it represents. In December 2020, only 66 per cent of the populations of 11 OECD countries indicated a willingness to be vaccinated. This had risen to 76 per cent by February 2021. The data from France, Germany and the US indicated that over a quarter of the population would refuse the vaccine. Vaccine hesitancy was age related, with more than half of 25- to 34-year-olds in France and one-third in the Netherlands indicating they would probably or definitely not be vaccinated.

UK data published by the Office for National Statistics (ONS) outlined clear areas of vaccine hesitancy. In July 2021, vaccine hesitancy rates in the UK were among the lowest in Europe, with only 4 per cent of adults reporting hesitancy. However the rates were higher among young people (11 per cent of those aged 16–17 being hesitant), ethnic minorities, with 21 per cent of Black adults and 14 per cent of Muslim adults being hesitant, among adults living in deprived areas (8 per cent) and those who were unemployed (12 per cent) (ONS, 2021a). These data on expressions of vaccine hesitancy were reflected in actual vaccination behaviours. In the UK on 29 September 2021, 89.5 per cent of the adult population had the first vaccination and 82.5 per cent both doses (Gov.UK, 2021b). The vaccination rates for ethnic minority groups aged 50 and over were lower than White British people of the same age (ONS, 2021b). In April 2021, 93.7 per cent of White British people aged over 50 had had a first dose of the vaccine compared with 66.8 per cent of Black Caribbeans and 71.2 per cent of Black Africans. In terms of socio-economic factors, 93.1 per cent of those working in higher administrative and professional occupations had had a first dose compared with 77.1 per cent of those who were long-term unemployed (ONS 2021b).

There has been speculation on the causes of vaccine hesitancy, especially mistrust of the state and of preventative technologies (OECD, 2021). However, actual evidence on its causes are more limited. One of the few studies to explore COVID-vaccine hesitancy and its link to risk perception was undertaken by Caserotti and her colleagues (2021), based on a questionnaire survey of 2,267 Italians recruited mainly from northern Italy shortly before, during and after the first Italian lockdown (March–July 2020). They found that intentions to be vaccinated were influenced by perceptions of the danger and by trust in vaccine technology: 'the more doubtful people are about vaccines in general, the less willing they were to get vaccinated, no matter the specific vaccine' (Caserotti et al, 2021, p. 7).

While research on receptiveness to warnings and other public health messages is limited, given the evidence that vaccine hesitancy is linked to social factors such as age, ethnicity and deprivation, social relations clearly plays a role. An article reflecting on vaccination at English Premier Division clubs provides some insights. Cunningham observes that while all players and staff at a few clubs, Wolves, Leeds, Brentford, Southampton, were fully vaccinated, at others coverage was more limited. This patchiness was a product of factions within the clubs: 'dressing rooms are like "mini-families" – close-knit groups with parental figures that quickly react to situations – that once a position is taken it is quickly entrenched. Where anti-vax theories have taken hold, it's proving hard to break them, particularly if leadership figures are involved' (Cunningham, 2021, p. 55).

Risk implications

In analysing the impact of risk messaging, it is easier to focus on and gain evidence on the nature of messages and their sources. While the clarity of the message and the trustworthiness of the messenger are clearly important, they do not explain how and why some individuals and groups are willing to listen to and act on warnings whereas others mistrust both warnings and their source. The responses both of individuals and groups appear to be shaped by cultural factors, especially how much individuals and groups share values and perceptions with those providing the warnings. Psychologists have termed this the 'White Male Effect' (Finucane et al, 2000).

Comment

In the early stages of the pandemic, there were major uncertainties about the new virus, how virulent it was, how it spread and how dangerous it was. Those countries that initially framed COVID-19 as a dangerous SARS- or Ebola-like disease that was both highly contagious and potentially lethal not only provided early warnings to their populations but could also be more consistent in their messaging. In contrast, those countries that initially framed COVID-19 as a milder flu-like disease had a greater challenge. Initially, they reassured their populations that there was no great danger. But as the disease spread, and it became clear that it was not only highly contagious but also dangerous, especially for vulnerable individuals, they had to change the message.

During the pandemic, governments had to meet the challenge of communicating complex scientific and epidemiological concepts in such a way that they could be understood and accepted by the population, resulting in behavioural changes that limited or stopped the spread of the virus. In different ways and for rather different reasons, Taiwan, Japan and New Zealand managed to do this successfully. In the UK and US, the messaging was undermined by the lack of a clear risk framework, a failure to punish leaders or their followers for breaches of the rules, and tensions between leaders and the scientific community. In New Zealand, surveys indicated that trust in the government was high, especially during the first wave (91 per cent trusted the government to manage the pandemic), though it did decline to 82 per cent in the summer, probably reflecting the impact of renewed clusters of the virus (New Zealand Herald, 2020). In the UK, a survey suggests that 57 per cent of those surveyed did not trust the government to control the spread of COVID-19, as the government's response was confused and inconsistent (Sky News, 2020).

PART II

Mitigating risk through science and technology

5

'Following the science': expertise and risk

Using experts and expertise to identify and manage risk

Governments in modern democratic societies accept that one of their primary roles is to protect their citizens. As the inquiry into the failure of the UK government to prevent BSE infecting humans noted most of the public believe that it is the government's role to minimise the hazards they are exposed to and 'the Government should do all that is reasonably practicable to see that the food that they eat and the medicines that they take are reasonably safe' (BSE Inquiry, 2000, para 1291). To provide such protection, the government needs to draw on experts' knowledge to identify the risks and decide how to mitigate them (HM Treasury, 2005, p. 45).

In normal times, this process tends to take place behind closed doors and attracts relatively little media and public attention. However during the COVID-19 pandemic, experts took on a more prominent and public role. In making decisions that impacted on the lives of all citizens, often in quite novel ways, politicians claimed to be 'following the science', and experts often legitimated these decisions, endorsing them in public forums such as televised briefings.

The institutional structure of science and scientists

Scientists play a key role in developing the knowledge and technologies that underpin modern societies. They work in a variety of settings, ranging from commercial enterprises such as pharmaceutical companies to charities and government-funded institutions, especially universities.

Low- and middle-income countries

Despite the limitations of government funding and institutional infrastructures, some countries have either developed their own specialist institutions or collaborated in multinational institutions.

Nigeria, one of the largest and most populous African countries, has a well-developed university sector and its own public health centre, the Nigeria Centre for Disease Control and Prevention (2022). This was established in 2011, being supported by the Federal Ministry of Health and other state bodies together with international partners. During the pandemic, the Nigerian CDC issued guidance on COVID-19 infection control for all health-care workers, managers and infection control teams as well as more general advice to the public.

Liberia was one of the three West African countries most affected by the Ebola epidemic (Honigsbaum, 2020). Following that epidemic, it established National Public Health Institute Liberia to bring together scientific expertise and to prepare for future epidemics (NPHIL, 2021). NPHIL issued advice and guidance on COVID-19.

Given limited resources in low- to middle-income countries, they often supplemented local scientific resources with international collaboration, drawing on regional and global resources. In Africa, the Africa Centres for Disease Control and Prevention, located in Addis Ababa, was launched in 2017. This technical institution is funded by the African Union and provides support for member states in detecting, controlling and responding to the threat of disease (Africa CDC, 2021a). Its aims include establishing early warning systems to identify health threats and natural disasters, and supporting or conducting regional and country hazard mapping and risk assessments (Africa CDC, 2021a). It published guidance on COVID-19 and preventive measures such as mask wearing and good hygiene.

Policy makers and scientists in low- and middle-income countries can draw on resources in high-income countries through collaboration or through accessing multinational agencies such as the WHO. In collaboration, researchers in low- and middle-income countries are likely to be 'down-stream'. For example, in the development of COVID-19 vaccines, the 'up-stream' hi-tech research and development took place in university and drug company laboratories mainly in Europe, East Asia and North America, and 'down-stream' clinical trials included those in low- and middle-income countries. The Africa CDC review of COVID-19 research identified 11 principal researchers engaged in drug and vaccine trials, mostly located in Kenya (Africa CDC, 2021b, p. 13).

Multinational agencies provide low- and middle-income countries with access to resources, including knowledge. The WHO is a United Nations agency that promotes global health. As high-income countries have the resources and health-care systems to provide universal health coverage for their populations, the WHO has focused on extending such coverage globally (WHO, 1978). It draws on funding, mainly from high-income countries, to develop ways of promoting global health. Thus, in collaboration with and mainly funded by the French government, the WHO has established a WHO Academy Campus in the biomedical district of Lyon in the south of France that supports medical researchers from low- and middle-income countries (WHO, 2021b).

High-income countries

High-income countries invest in scientific research. In 2017, total medical and health research funding in the US was $182.3 billion, with industry contributing 67 per cent of the total ($121.8 billion) (Research America, 2018).

Such funding supports scientists and their research in a diversity of settings (pharmaceutical companies, university departments and research institutes) and in a variety of disciplines. While scientists compete for funding, they do so within specific scientific communities – groups of scientists who share an interest in the same topics and/or academic disciplines. Such communities cross national boundaries and include media through which their members can interact and share their interests; these include learned societies, conferences, journals and increasingly groups based on apps. There is often an internal hierarchy in these communities, with senior established members playing a lead role.

The interaction between scientists and policy makers

Low- and middle-income countries

Medical and scientific communities tend to be small in size and usually located in major urban centres, often in close proximity to policy makers. If there is mutual confidence, then there can be close informal interaction, with government policy making being informed by expert advice. In Senegal, following the Ebola epidemic, the government set up a Health Emergency Operations Centre, which brought together medical expertise as a resource to respond to future epidemics. The government appointed Dr Abdoulaye Bousso, a doctor specialising in orthopaedic and trauma surgery with expertise in disaster management and health emergencies, to direct the centre (El Daif, 2021). In March 2020, the Senegalese Ministry of Health alerted the centre when the first case was identified, and acted on its director's advice as it prepared for the epidemic (El Daif, 2021).

In Tanzania, President John Magaufuli was sceptical about medical advice. At the start of the pandemic, when doctors and others were warning about unexplained deaths, including those of senior politicians, Magaufuli, influenced by religious leaders, denied the existence of the virus. He replaced the permanent secretary of the health ministry with a COVID-19 denier, Dr Mchembe (Odour, 2021). When President Magaufuli died on 17 March 2021 (probably of COVID-19), he was replaced by Ms Samia Suluhu Hassan, who was receptive to expert advice. She sacked Dr Mchembe, appointed expert epidemiological advisers and allowed the ministry to issue science-based guidelines, advocating the wearing of masks and the use of PPE by health workers. She wore a face mask on her official visit to Uganda in April 2021 (Bariyo, 2021).

High-income countries

Scientific communities are large and complex, and are dispersed throughout national and regional centres. In the US, the federal government funds a network of medical research units, the National Institutes for Health (NIH). Within the NIH, the National Institute of Allergy and Virology (NIAV) conducts and supports a programme of research into infectious diseases, influenza and vaccine development. Anthony Fauci was its director from 1984; he had access to and could make available scientific evidence relevant to an understanding of SARS-CoV-2 (Abutaleb and Paletta, 2021, pp 153–5). The federal government also funds a major public health programme, the CDC. This monitors threats to the health and safety of the US and provides advice and guidance on protection of the country's citizens. Its director, Robert Redfield, was appointed by Donald Trump in 2018 (Abutaleb and Paletta, 2021, pp 65–71).

While both the NIAV and CDC are federally funded, they operate independently from federal government. Both communicate research findings and health advice directly to the public. During the COVID-19 pandemic, the CDC regularly published guidance and advice to the public on who was at-risk (CDC, 2020a), the similarities and difference between COVID-19 and flu (CDC, 2021a) and the benefits of getting a COVID-19 vaccination (CDC, 2021d).

At the start of the pandemic, there was no formal mechanism in the US for the executive to regularly consult key scientists. In the early stages of the pandemic, the president had ad hoc briefings. On 23 January, when the Chinese authorities announced a lockdown in the city of Wuhan, the president was briefed by his chief security briefer that the new disease was 'Just like flu. We don't think it's as deadly as SARS' (Woodward, 2020a, p. 230).

As the pandemic developed in late January 2020, these ad hoc briefings were replaced with a more formal structure, the White House Coronavirus Task Force. Initially, it was chaired by Alex Azur, the Secretary of Health and Human Services, and brought together health and national security experts with key policy makers to discuss the repatriation of US citizens from China. By the end of February, the president was concerned that his administration's response to the pandemic was not inspiring public confidence. He replaced Azur with Mike Pence, the vice president, bringing the Task Force into the White House (Gerstein, 2020, p. 170). Following Task Force meetings, there was usually a press briefing led by the president. If Trump approved the Task Force recommendations, they formed the basis of his scripted speech, though he often ad libbed and went 'off message'. From the start of the pandemic there were contradictory messages, optimistic from the president and more cautious from his advisers (Cathey, 2020).

Deborah Birx played a key role in persuading the president to accept lockdown on 16 March 2020. She was a highly experienced medical researcher, and early in the pandemic she had returned from her work leading US AIDS relief in Africa to provide advice to the Task Force and president. She was convinced that US policy and risk messaging needed to change (Abutaleb and Paletta, 2021, pp 134–42). Using her contacts in Europe, she obtained comprehensive data on the rapid spread of the virus, especially in Italy. Given the lack of testing in the US, there was a lack of data, but it was clear from outbreaks on cruise ships, in care homes and in the community that the virus was both highly infectious and taking hold. Based on the European data, Birx was able to show that the US was likely to experience an exponential rise in infections and subsequent deaths (Abutaleb and Paletta, 2021, pp 121–30).

Trump did initially accept the advice to lockdown, but he quickly tried to reverse the decision. On 17 April, in the middle of a supposed 30-day extension of the US lockdown, he voiced opposition to the lockdown, tweeting 'Liberate Minnesota', 'Liberate Michigan' and 'Liberate Virginia' (Woodward, 2020a, p. 353). This was a sign of major tension and conflict between the president, his inner circle of advisers and medical experts. In the early summer, for example, the CDC was advising the public to wear masks (CDC, 2020b), while the president was not following his administration's own guidance.

The relationship between Trump and his inner circle and medical experts such as Fauci, Redfield and Birx was tense. Trump wanted to control the message about COVID-19. He felt that the public health messaging was undermining his campaign for re-election. Trump and his colleagues exerted pressure on Redfield to minimise the risks and Hahn (Commissioner of the Food and Drug Administration) to approve untested treatments (Abutaleb and Paletta, 2021, pp 288–91). The key scientists, Fauci, Birx, Redfield and Hahn, responded by forming an informal alliance. They decided to meet regularly, to defend each other if criticised and to counter lies and mistruths. Birx, Redfield and Hahn were political appointees, so could be fired, and they made it known that if one of them was fired then the other two would resign (Abutaleb and Paletta, 2021, pp 291–4).

Despite pressure from the White House to minimise public health measures and to approve untested treatments for COVID-19, for the most part the scientific community remained intact and protected its independence. Fauci, in particular, acquired the status of a media celebrity, enabling him to continue communicating in a hostile environment and to claim that science was independent. When asked about his response to people 'who might think you have a political agenda', he commented: 'The common enemy is the virus. So, it really doesn't make any sense if you have a political divide about whether you should be wearing a mask or not. It has nothing at all to do with politics' (Hackel, 2020).

In the UK, a general election was not due until 2024. While Trump tried to change scientific opinion to suit his optimistic messages, Prime Minister Boris Johnson claimed to be 'following the science', especially when justifying unpopular decisions. When announcing his decision to effectively cancel Christmas celebrations at the end of 2020, Boris Johnson noted that the emerging evidence on a 'new variant, and the potential risks it poses' meant that 'we cannot continue with Christmas as planned' and that 'we have said throughout this pandemic that we must and we will be guided by the science. When the science changes, we must change our response. When the virus changes its method of attack, we must change our method of defence' (Johnson, 2020d).

As in the US, the UK had well-funded medical and public health institutes. However, there were important differences in the ways in which this funding was allocated. With the exception of the direct funding of Public Health England, most funding is channelled through research institutes located mainly in universities and the NHS. The UK established a National Institute for Health and Care Research (NIHR) (NIHR, 2022) in 2006, but compared with the US's NIH its funding is limited.

Given the dispersion of scientific expertise in universities and research centres, the UK government has two main mechanisms for accessing the expertise it needs: directly employing scientific advisers and inviting scientists to sit on a range of advisory committees. The key scientific advisors at the start of the pandemic were the UK's Chief Medical Officer, Chris Whitty, and his four deputies, including Jonathan Van-Tam and Dr Jenny Harries and the CSA, Sir Patrick Vallance. Whitty is a public health expert, an epidemiologist and a former professor at the London School of Hygiene and Tropical Medicine. When he was CSA at the Department of International Development, he played a key role in the UK's response to the West African Ebola outbreak (Gov.UK, 2021c). Dr Harries is a career public health doctor who had a vital position in the UK's response to various epidemics, including Ebola, Zika, monkeypox and MERS. During the pandemic, she took on two new roles, becoming Chief Executive of the UK Health Security Agency, an agency that replaced Public Health England on 1 April 2021, and Head of NHS Track and Trace (Gov.UK, 2021d). Sir Patrick Vallance has been the UK government's CSA since 2018. He has a medical background: for 20 years he worked as a doctor and medical researcher, with a professorship at University College London. He then joined a drug company, GlaxoSmithKline, leading their research and development.

These expert advisers provide policy makers with access to expert advice and are supported by a network of expert committees (see Table 5.1, Gov.UK, 2021e).

This network is extensive, I have included two SAGE subgroups in Table 5.1. There are nine in total. In normal times, these committees operate behind

Table 5.1: The network of advisory committees providing expert advice to policy makers in the UK

Acronym	Full title	General Role	Role in pandemic	Chair	Membership
COBRA/ COBR	Civil Contingencies Committee (The acronym derives from Cabinet Office Briefing Room A)	Committee that responds to major threats to security in the UK that are considered national emergencies and threaten major disruption	Regular meetings from the start of the pandemic to assess the threat of COVID-19	Normally the prime minister, but he was absent for first five pandemic meetings and some subsequent meetings	Relevant ministers and officials
SAGE	Scientific Advisory Group for Emergencies	The group provides scientific and technical advice to policy makers during emergencies. It works alongside COBRA and was first used to provide advice in the 2009 swine flu (H1N1) epidemic	Following the first COVID-19 meeting on 22 January 2020, SAGE met regularly to collate scientific evidence on the spread of the virus and to consider the best ways to protect the population and services	During the pandemic, SAGE was co-chaired by the CMO (Chris Whitty) and the CSA (Sir Patrick Vallance)	Its membership depends on the nature of the emergency. During the pandemic, it included over 70 participants: key experts advisers and senior academics in epidemiology, virology, clinicians, behavioural scientists and data scientists
SPI-M	Scientific Pandemic Influenza Group on Modelling	This group provides expert advice to SAGE on infectious disease modelling and epidemiology	By monitoring epidemiological evidence, modellers provided predictions of rates of infection, impact on hospitals and death rates	The membership list does not identify the chair but the Deputy CMO, Jonathan Van-Tam, is a member of the group and is likely to have played a key role	The membership (80+) draws on research teams who have an established record of modelling and predicting the spread of infectious disease, and the impact of mitigating measures

(continued)

Table 5.1: The network of advisory committees providing expert advice to policy makers in the UK (continued)

Acronym	Full title	General Role	Role in pandemic	Chair	Membership
SPI-B	Independent Scientific Pandemic Insights Group on Behaviours	This group provides advice to SAGE on individual and collective behaviour in response to the risk of infectious disease	This group provided advice on how the population is likely to respond to measures to mitigate risks such as social distancing measures	The membership list does not identify the chair	The membership (40+) includes behavioural scientists such as Professor Reicher and Professor Michie as well as members of the Cabinet Office's Behavioural Insights Team (Nudge Unit)
NERVTAG	New and Emerging Respiratory Virus Threats Advisory Group	This group provides expert advice to the CMO on the risks of new and emerging respiratory viruses, including SARS-CoV-2. It replaced the Scientific Advisory Group on Pandemic Influenza (SPI) in 2014	This group provided scientific risk assessment and mitigation advice	Professor Sir Peter Horby, Professor of Emerging Infectious Diseases at the University of Oxford.	The membership (18) includes leading scientists in clinical medicine, virology, epidemiology, vaccinology and bio-statistical modelling. There is some overlap with other committees, and six additional members were co-opted for COVID-19
JCVI	Joint Committee on Vaccination and Immunisation	The committee advises all UK government health departments on vaccination	The committee reviewed the evidence on the safety and efficacy of all COVID-19 vaccines and advised on how, when and to whom these vaccines should be given	Professor Andrew Pollard chaired the committee before the pandemic, but given his involvement in the development of the Oxford vaccine he recused himself, and was replaced by Professor Lim Wen Shem	Normally 20 members, mainly with vaccine, immunology and virology expertise, plus a lay member and public health representatives. During the pandemic, a subcommittee (15) provided additional advice

closed doors, though some provide regular public updates on risks. Since 2015, the New and Emerging Respiratory Virus Threats Advisory Group (NERVTAG) has produced annual reports warning of the dangers of new respiratory viruses. These have been acknowledged by government but attracted limited media and public attention. Van-Tam, the first chair of NERVTAG, wrote in the foreword to the first annual report:

> In the post pandemic [2009 A(H1N1) 'swine flu'] we have seen further emerging respiratory virus threats with potential consequences for humans; Influenza A(H7N9), A(H5N8) and A(H5N6) and the Middle East Respiratory Syndrome coronavirus (MERS CoV). We are reminded that we cannot predict the future, beyond saying that another pandemic is inevitable at some point... (NERVTAG, 2015, p. 5)

During the pandemic, both the scientific advisers and scientific committees became more visible; indeed, some developed media profiles. Whitty, Van-Tam and Vallance all featured regularly in the media. SAGE and JCVI reports and recommendations and guidelines were reported and discussed in the media.

The UK avoided the open war between scientists and policy makers that characterised the US while Trump was president. However, given the poor performance of the UK compared with other high-income countries, and given its well-developed scientific base and mechanisms for accessing scientific knowledge, critics have identified shortcomings:

- 'Following the science', and the failure of policy makers to take the initiative: While science can help policy makers understand risks and how they can be mitigated, it does not make the decisions. Policy makers in the UK used science to avoid or delay making decisions and did not critically challenge or seek to interrogate the science. The failure of policy makers to provide leadership was reflected in their continued use and dependence on SAGE. At the start of most national crises, SAGE meets to enable policy makers to gain an overview of the challenge and how it can be met. Ministers and their departments then take over the response. In the case of the COVID-19 pandemic, this takeover did not happen: SAGE continued to meet. Sasse, Haddon and Nice (2020) note that an over-reliance on SAGE resulted in delayed decision making that was especially damaging at the start of the pandemic: 'At times the prime minister and ministers waited until the scientific evidence was overwhelming rather than using it alongside other inputs to make their own judgements' (p. 5).
  There was also a failure to use COBRA effectively. It should act as a forum for key policy makers, drive policy and make request specific scientific

inputs from SAGE. It failed to do this. One member of SAGE described COBRA as a 'void of decision making' at the centre of government at the start of the pandemic (Haddon, 2021). The failure of the prime minister to attend the first five COVID-19 COBRA meetings reflected the low priority he gave to COVID-19 at the start of the pandemic.

- The role of key scientific advisers: This is challenging, as these advisers effectively act as intermediaries between the scientific community and policy makers. Sasse, Haddon and Nice (2020) observe that scientific advisers did not 'sell out' to policy makers but may have self-censored. Perhaps this was most evident at the start of the pandemic when there were uncertainties about the transmissibility and lethalness of the virus. In early March, Jenny Harries, at the time Deputy CMO, justified the decision not to reduce social interactions by closing schools and cancelling sports events, arguing that these measures were not supported by science. She observed that 'The virus will not survive very long outside' and that 'Many outdoor events, particularly, are relatively safe' (BBC, 2020c). Given the very different conclusion that Birx in the US arrived at, using the same data at the same time, it is difficult to understand how Harries reached these conclusions.

  The scientific advisers were placed in a compromised position when Dominic Cummings broke the lockdown rules. Sir Patrick Vallance avoided commenting, saying he did not want to get involved in politics, while Jonathan Van-Tam was clear in his condemnation, stating that 'In my opinion the rules are clear ... they are for the benefit of all. In my opinion they apply to all' (Parveen, 2020b).

- Narrowness and limitations of the scientific advice: The key science advisers and committee members represent the elite of the UK's scientific community. However, this elite is drawn from a small section of the scientific community. For example, the membership of SAGE has been criticised as being 'dominated by too narrow a group of medical scientists and modellers at the expense of others such as external public health experts' (Sasse, Haddon and Nice, 2020, p. 7). The House of Commons Committee on Science and Technology commented on the membership of SAGE, observing that 'there was a particular reliance on epidemiological expertise at the beginning of SAGE's operation – reflecting the paucity of data early in the pandemic – and identifying an apparent gap in the provision of independent advice on non-medical impacts' (House of Commons, Science and Technology Committee, 2021, p. 4). The narrow range of expertise meant that advisers focused on health risks and tended not to consider other risks. For example, the lack of economists in SAGE and other committees meant that decisions about economic issues were made separately in the Treasury, and the interaction between health and economic risks was not considered. For example, the Chancellor of the Exchequer funded a scheme to stimulate the hospitality sector in the summer of 2020, Eat Out to Help Out, which contributed to the second wave of infection in the UK (Sasse, Haddon and Nice, 2020, p. 6).

This narrowness was also evident in the membership and function of the JCVI. Its membership was mainly drawn from scientists with expertise in virology, immunisation and the development of vaccines, yet this committee was asked to provide advice on the priorities for the vaccination programme, raising complex social and ethical issues that were outside the competence of most committee members. When considering whether COVID-19 vaccines should be offered to children aged 12–15, the committee avoided making a recommendation passing the decision back to the UK's CMOs (Gov.UK, 2021f).

- Pressure on scientists and the dangers of burnout: During the pandemic, scientists were asked to undertake new activities and were subject to pressures that were beyond their normal remit. They had to set aside their normal work to deliver reports to short deadlines and in forms accessible to policy makers, and they were often in the media spotlight. An early victim of this pressure was Professor Neil Ferguson, whose report on the likely outcome of the first wave of COVID-19 contributed to the first UK lockdown (Ferguson et al, 2020). On 6 May 2020, the media reported that he had resigned from SAGE as he had breached lockdown rules when a woman visited him at his home. He accepted he had made an error of judgement (BBC, 2020g). In November 2021, Sir Jeremy Farrar, an eminent medical scientist and Director of the Wellcome Trust, resigned from SAGE. In his resignation statement, he acknowledged that SAGE had provided the government with vital expert evidence, but often under huge pressure. He had considered resigning in September 2020 when 'I began to question the point of giving advice to a body [the government] that chose not to use it' (Cookson, 2021). Although he made it clear that his resignation was to concentrate on his role with the Wellcome Trust, it was also evident that he was critical of the government's over-reliance on vaccination. He advocated a 'vaccine plus' strategy that would include mask-wearing on public transport and in shops and indoor spaces, as well as increased ventilation and flexible working (Cookson, 2021).

- Lack of transparency: Given policy makers claimed to be 'following the science' when making policy decisions that had major impacts on people's everyday lives, it was important that those affected by these decisions understood how and why they were made. For the public to trust 'the science', there needs to be transparency. At the start of the pandemic, there were low levels of transparency. As the Science and Technology Committee noted, 'there were initial delays in the publication of SAGE evidence, minutes and the disclosure of expert advisers' (House of

Commons, Science and Technology Committee, 2021, p. 4). Sasse, Haddon and Nice (2020) argue that the government's failure to be open about scientific advice at the start of the pandemic undermined public confidence and 'also undermined the implementation of specific policies: for instance, making it harder for parents and teachers to have confidence in the government's plan to reopen schools' (Sasse, Haddon and Nice, 2020, p. 7).

Comment

In high-income countries with established universities and research centres, there is substantial scientific expertise regarding the nature and transmission of infectious diseases and their impacts on individuals and communities. Different countries have developed different mechanisms to mobilise this expertise. In the US, the NIAV and CDC provide national and global resources. In the early stages of the pandemic Donald Trump drew on this expertise in his White House team, but he also drew on 'alternative' expertise. In the UK at the start of the pandemic, there was no equivalent to the NIAV and CDC, and their function was replicated by a complex network of expert committees in which some scientific groups were better represented than others. Policy makers favoured some scientific voices; for example, bio- and medical scientists tended to dominate the UK advisory network.

Case Study 6: Droplet versus aerosol spray: conflicting scientific opinion on the mode of transmission of SARS-CoV-2

Given the uncertainties associated with the novel SARS-CoV-2 virus, scientific knowledge appeared to offer policy makers and the public a degree of certainty. Trusting the knowledge provided by scientists, policy makers and the public could bridge the chasm of their ignorance and allow them to take actions that would minimise the risks of the new disease (Möllering, 2001). This trust was based on the belief that there was undisputed scientific knowledge based on scientific research. In this case study, I examine the ways in which scientific knowledge was shaped by relationships in scientific communities and between these communities and policy makers. I explore the ways in which knowledge about the transmission of the virus was constructed and shaped policy.

At the start of the pandemic, the dominant view among medical researchers was that the virus was spread by droplets, and with the exception of Japan, this view was accepted by policy makers in most countries. There was an alternative theory that aerosol spray played a key role in transmission, and that transmission could be interrupted by measures such as mask wearing and ventilation. This theory was based on research by scientists outside the core medical/clinical community and was initially dismissed as lacking evidence, but over time became the accepted orthodoxy.

Identifying and managing the risk of infection

At the start of the pandemic, it was clear that COVID-19 was caused by a virus that infected the human respiratory system, but how it entered that system was not clear. There were two possibilities:

- Droplet transmission by coughing, sneezing or singing: an infected person could breathe out droplets containing the virus that people standing close by could breathe in. Such droplets, being relatively heavy, could settle on nearby surfaces and be transferred if someone touched the surface and then touched their mouth or eyes (formite transmission). If droplets and formites were the main route of transmission, then the most effective hygienic measures were keeping at least 2 metres away from other people, covering coughs and sneezes, washing hands regularly and disinfecting surfaces.
- Aerosol transmission by breathing, coughing or sneezing: an infected person would spray aerosol (micro-droplets containing the virus) into the air. This aerosol could hang in the air for some time, especially in confined spaces, infecting people who entered these spaces some time later. The most effective ways to limit aerosol transmission were to improve ventilation where possible, to avoid crowded places, especially poorly ventilated ones, and to wear some form of face covering or mask.

Evidence from the 2003 SARS epidemic

In the early stages of the pandemic, there was uncertainty about how SARS-CoV-2 was transmitted. However, it was clear that the new virus was a coronavirus like SARS, so it was possible that it was transmitted in the same way. The 2003 SARS outbreak had been relatively short-lived and rapidly contained, but it had been closely scrutinised, especially in Hong Kong (Honigsbaum, 2020, 167–182).

In Hong Kong, there had been several superspreading events at the Metropole Hotel and Block E of the Amoy Gardens buildings. At the Metropole, Professor Liu from Guangzhou checked into room 911 on 21 February 2003. The following morning, he was admitted to the Kwong Wah hospital, where he died on 4 March from SARS. A further 17 people at the hotel contracted SARS. Within 72 hours, some of these guests had travelled to seven other countries, and there were superspreading events in Hanoi (63 cases), Toronto (136 cases) and Singapore (195 cases) (Whaley, 2006a, pp 41–8).

On 14 March, Mr LTC, a 33-year-old man with autoimmune kidney disease, was staying with his brother in Block E of the Amoy Gardens buildings when he developed a fever and had diarrhoea. On 26 March 2003, 15 residents were admitted to hospital. By 31 March, 213 residents from the building had been admitted with symptoms of SARS. Most of these (107) were from two floors, 7 and 8, on Block E. In all, 329 residents of Amoy Gardens Buildings were infected, and 42 died (Whaley, 2006b, p. 157).

The outbreaks in Hong Kong were investigated by the Hong Kong Department of Health and by environmental health experts from the WHO (Whaley, 2006a, p. 147). The WHO team observed that aerosol transmission was the most likely route of infection. Rooms in the hotels were pressurised so 'infected aerosol would not enter from the corridor'. It was unlikely that heavier droplets were involved as there was no evidence of droplet contamination on surfaces such as the lift, door handles and handrail; nor were guests on other floors and hotel staff infected (Whaley, 2006a, p. 147). The WHO team investigating the outbreak at the Amoy Gardens Buildings noted that a combination of factors accounted for the superspreading event there: the index case had a high viral load in his faeces, the bathroom drains had been removed or dried out in many flats, and many residents had fitted powerful fans in their bathroom that sucked in air from the waste system. The team concluded that the virus had been carried by aerosol or droplets between flats (Whaley, 2006b).

Given the lack of material deposited on surfaces, it seemed probable that the primary route of transmission in the Hong Kong superspreading events was by aerosol spray, 'droplets of infectious material ... sufficiently small to remain almost indefinitely airborne and to be transmitted long distances' (Tang et al, 2006).

The debate about the transmission of SARS-CoV-2

Despite the evidence from the 2003 SARS epidemic that aerosol spray could play a key role in transmission of coronavirus, there was debate among scientists about how the new virus was transmitted and the most effective way of interrupting this transmission. With the exception of Japan, the dominant scientific view was that droplets were the main route of transmission.

Early in the pandemic, researchers in Japan identified the importance of aerosol transmission. As noted in Chapter 4, in March 2020, the Japanese government adopted its 3C approach, highlighting the importance of good ventilation to disperse aerosol (Government of Japan, 2020). The research in Japan drew on studies of the transmission of COVID-19 on board a cruise ship quarantined in Yokohama in February 2020 (Kakimoto et al, 2020), epidemiological analysis of clusters of cases (Greenhalgh et al, 2021) and computer simulation of aerosol spray. Makoto Tsubokura, a researcher at the

Computational Fluid Dynamics lab at Kobe University and the government institute RIKEN, used a supercomputer to simulate the spread of airborne transmission in trains, offices, schools, hospitals and other public spaces. The simulation indicated that when people sneezed or coughed, or just talked, they emitted small particles that hung in the air for hours, even days. He concluded that the best way of preventing spread was to ensure air circulated and use (well-fitted) masks (Craft, 2020). Greenhalgh and her colleagues (2021b) noted that in Japan, Hitoshi Oshitani, a virologist, played a key role in identifying the main mode of transmission. He worked with a professor of mathematics to identify and analyse early clusters, finding that most transmission was through superspreading events – this indicating that aerosol played a key role in transmission.

Outside Japan, the initial scientific and policy makers' consensus was that heavier droplets were the main medium of transmission, so the main thrust of prevention was on hygienic measures that interrupted transmission. There was no general support for measures that focused on aerosol transmission, such as ventilation or mask wearing.

The orthodox view that the virus was transmitted by droplets and formites was evident in WHO documents. In a scientific brief published on 7 March 2020, the WHO (2020e) highlighted the role of droplets and direct contact transmission of the virus:

> According to current evidence, COVID-19 virus is transmitted between people through respiratory droplets and contact routes. Droplet transmission occurs when a person is in in close contact (within 1 m) with someone who has respiratory symptoms (e.g. coughing or sneezing). … Droplet transmission may also occur through fomites in the immediate environment around the infected person. Therefore, transmission of the COVID-19 virus can occur by direct contact with infected people and indirect contact with surfaces in the immediate environment or with objects used on the infected person (e.g. stethoscope or thermometer). (WHO, 2020e)

The scientific brief acknowledged that aerosol transmission was possible, but noted that there was no reported evidence from China of such transmission. The brief noted but did not reference research indicating that airborne transmission was possible, although it stated 'These initial findings need to be interpreted carefully' (WHO, 2020e). The brief stated that if aerosol transmission took place, it would probably be associated with invasive medical procedures such as intubation (WHO, 2020e). On 28 February 2020, the WHO issued a video that identified droplets as the main mode of transmission, and advocated cleaning surfaces and hand washing to prevent transmission (WHO, 2020b, viewed 8 million times).

In July 2020, 239 scientists signed a letter to the WHO and other health agencies highlighting the role of microdroplets (aerosol) in the transmission of SARS-CoV-2 (Morowska and Milton, 2020). In response to this letter, the WHO issued a further scientific briefing. This grudgingly accepted the possibility of aerosol transmission, but dismissed epidemiological evidence of aerosol spread in indoor settings – noting that there were alternative explanations for the findings (WHO, 2020c).

The consensus view was also evident in national and regional responses. In the Canadian province of British Columbia, the public health messaging at the start of the pandemic stressed the role of droplet transmission. For example, a tweet by the province's Centre for Disease Control included a video with the statement that 'the new #coronavirus is spread by droplets that come from the mouth or nose. The droplets don't stay floating in the air. This is not an airborne virus' (Greenhalgh et al, 2021). Despite pressure from unions representing workers in health care for measures to restrict aerosol transmission, the health agencies were unwilling to act. Dr Henry, the provincial health officer, was dismissive. She suggested it was 'a tempest in a teapot' (Lindsay, 2020), claiming there was a consensus that the virus was spread mainly through large droplets and 'It's not transmitted long distances in the air column. We're all on the same page about that' (Lindsay, 2020). In January 2021, the British Columbian Nursing Union (BCNU) claimed success in its campaign to get the British Columbian CDC to recognise aerosol transmission, so they could gain protection with improved PPE. In its revised guidelines, the British Columbian CDC did not use the term aerosol, but referred to 'smaller droplets', noting that these were light, could float in the air longer and collect in enclosed spaces, resulting in COVID-19 infections (BCNU, 2021).

Why was there resistance to the aerosol theory?

Greenhalgh and her colleagues (2021) examined how and why the voices of supporters of the aerosol theory were initially suppressed. They found that the most prestigious and externally recognised discipline at the start of the pandemic was infectious disease control, mostly involving clinicians who worked in hospitals. They observed that clinicians in this discipline were 'experts in topics such as wound management – for which droplet spread is predominant and hand washing is an effective intervention' (2021b). Senior members of the discipline had well-established links to key policy makers, acting as advisers and sitting on advisory committees, for example. Together with key policy makers such as Fauci in the US and Whitty and Vallance in the UK, they were members of the medical profession. Members of the discipline also claimed access to the best available evidence, that created by randomised control trials (RCTs) undertaken in clinical settings. Since

Table 5.2: Relative standing of supporters of aerosol and droplet theories

	Supporters of droplet theory	Supporters of aerosol theory
Discipline(s)	Clinicians working in infection control	Non-medical scientists, chemists and engineers
Linkages to policy makers	Well-established links with and shared background with key policy makers	Poor linkage with policy makers and no common background
Status of knowledge	Based on clinical experience and research	Based on theoretical analyses, supported by simulations plus epidemiological data

Archie Cochrane (1972) lambasted his medical colleagues for failing to base their practice on the best possible evidence, RCTs have become the gold standard of medical research and practice. Indeed, undertaking trials and assessing their effectiveness through systematic reviews has become a key and paradigmatic source of medical knowledge.

The researchers representing the dissenting voice, the supporters of aerosol diffusion, were mainly from non-medical disciplines such as chemistry and engineering. They were neither members of advisory committees nor involved in key decision-making networks. Their methods did not achieve medical gold standard specification. In the early stages of the pandemic, their aerosol theory was dismissed on the grounds that their methodologies were weak, 'their empirical findings ... untrustworthy or insignificant, and their contributions to debate ... unhelpful' (Greenhalgh et al, 2021; (see Table 5.2).

Risk implications

At the start of the pandemic, infectious disease experts were an insider group (Alaszewski and Brown, 2012. pp 89–113). They were co-opted into the policy-making process, ensuring that most policy makers accepted their claims that droplets were the main medium of virus transmission and that public health measures such as cleaning surfaces, personal hygiene and social distancing were the most effective ways of mitigating the risk of transmission. In contrast, the scientists supporting the dissenting view that the main route of transmission was by aerosol formed an outsider group, an alliance of researchers from different disciplines who did not have established relationship or informal contacts with policy makers. They had to use outsider tactics to make their voice heard; open letters, articles in journals and newspapers, and postings on social media, especially Twitter.

The outsider group did manage to shift the scientific consensus. The WHO withdrew its July 2020 Scientific Briefing (WHO, 2020c) and replaced it in December 2020 (WHO, 2020i) with a document advocating mask wearing, adding a document on 1 March 2021 (WHO, 2021c) stressing the importance of ventilation of spaces. The December 2020 document acknowledged the possibility of aerosol transmission, calling for more research and evidence. The March 2021 document drew on the 'outsider' disciplines through a panel of environment and engineering control experts and accepted the existence of aerosol transmission, focusing on ways to mitigate it (WHO, 2021c). In the UK, the shifting emphasis from droplet to aerosol transmission resulted in a public health campaign in November 2021 to 'stop covid-19 hanging about'. The campaign was accompanied by a film that demonstrated the ways in COVID-19 particles built up and lingered in an unventilated room, and how good ventilation would disperse these particles quickly (Gov.UK, 2021g).

The failure of policy makers to critically evaluate scientific evidence and acknowledge that aerosol spray was a major route of transmission had a number of negative effects:

- Delays in implementing effective measures to mitigate the risks of transmission: At the start of the pandemic, Japan identified aerosol spray as a major route of transmission and took action to counter it. Such action did not take place in the UK until some 18 months later.
- Lack of public awareness of the measures that could be taken to mitigate the risks of infection and transmission: An online survey of a representative sample of the population in the UK found that nearly two-thirds (64 per cent) of participants were unaware that ventilation could interrupt the transmission of COVID-19 and less than a third (29 per cent) were ventilating their home when they had visitors (Gov. UK, 2021g).
- Conspiracy theories were fuelled by the evidence that scientists didn't know how the virus was transmitted.

Comment

The relationship between science, policy and risk management in the pandemic was complex. Claims by key policy makers such as Boris Johnson that they were 'following the science' simplify what were complex relationships. As Mulkay (1979) makes clear in his study of scientific knowledge, the creation of scientific knowledge and its subsequent application is the product of social relations within scientific communities and between scientific communities and policy makers. Within scientific communities, knowledge is created through negotiations that involve social and technical resources. The acceptance of scientific knowledge by policy makers and in the wider community is shaped by the social standing of the scientist and the extent to which their 'knowledge' fits within pre-existing knowledge and perceptions.

'Following the science' implies that scientific knowledge provides an objective representation of the physical world and that rational action can be based on this. However, as is clear from Case Study 6 on droplet versus aerosol transmission, the dominant scientific consensus may not be the best representation of reality. Despite strong evidence that aerosol spray played an important role in the transmission of SARS, the initial consensus outside Japan was that larger droplets were more important, so transmission could be reduced by hygiene measures such as surface cleaning and hand sanitising. It was more than a year before most policy makers accepted that aerosol transmission was important and that measures such as mask wearing and improved ventilation could play an important role in prevention. The evidence was available, but policy makers did not seek it; nor did they question the advice they were being given.

The receptiveness of policy makers and the wider public to scientific knowledge was also shaped by social processes and, in particular during the pandemic, by the populist movements that shaped politics in many countries (I discuss this in Chapter 8, which considers conspiracy theories). As van der Molen and Brown (2021) observe in their study of responses to COVID-19 in the Netherlands, 'In "following the science", the centre-right cabinet has, of course, made political decisions in terms of which science, and which expert institutions, to heed' (p. 454). Populist leaders tended to be sceptical of 'experts' and reluctant to accept unpopular public health measures such as the lockdown of social and economic activities to prevent or reduce the spread of the virus. When they were forced to do so by rising infection and death rates, they did so reluctantly, and sought to remove restrictions as quickly as possible – thereby creating the conditions for new waves of infection.

Normally, negotiations within scientific communities and between scientific and policy communities are not visible; they take place behind closed doors. During the pandemic, given the major impact that some of the policy decisions had on the population, there was pressure to make the process more transparent, for example in the UK for the key advisory and decision-making committees to publish their advice and decisions. Such increased visibility makes it possible to identify the key participants and their interactions; as I have shown in Case Study 6, it is possible to identify the changing scientific consensus and its impact on policy making. Conflict and tensions tend to highlight the social processes and participants involved in a decision. It is more difficult to examine these relationships when there is consensus. For example in Chapter 3, I note the ways in which scientific experts on the JCVI in the UK made recommendations about vaccination priorities that had major social and ethical implications. The health minister was happy to endorse their decisions, emphasising that 'we are committed to vaccinating according to need' (Hancock, 2021b) and enabling him to avoid a discussion of the other possible goals of vaccination.

6

Risk work to maintain services during the pandemic

Risk issue: the disruptive effects of serious illnesses

All societies experience and manage disease and illness. While minor illnesses can be and usually are absorbed within the flow of everyday activities, serious illness is not: it creates uncertainty and threatens the continued existence of normal life. This disruption is managed differently in different situations.

Managing the disruption of serious illness: risk and other strategies

While illness is a universal phenomenon, responses to it vary: they are shaped by social processes, the ways in which people live and interact, and cultural factors, collective beliefs and knowledge. These differences can be seen by comparing the responses to illness in small-scale intimate societies with those in larger scale societies of strangers.

Small-scale intimate societies were the focus of anthropological study during the 20th century. In these societies, individuals live in close proximity. Interactions take place between those whose duties and obligations are defined by kinship relations (Givon and Young, 2001). This proximity and intimacy means that when an individual becomes ill, the disruption tends to spread through the whole community. Lewis (2000) observed the ways in which serious illness disrupted life in small rural villages in Northern Papua New Guinea: 'The spread of concern, the variety of constraints imposed on ordinary life – barriers to paths, a ban on dance and song, taboos on food or movement – the way they overcast and disrupted normal village life sometimes gave a public quality to the hidden suffering [of illness]' (Lewis, 2000, p. 80).

In intimate societies, responses to serious illness are shaped by cultural factors, especially beliefs about the ways in which natural and supernatural forces interact with individuals and communities. Coderey (2015), in a study of Buddhist villagers in Rakhine State, Western Myanmar, found that illness was perceived to be an ever-present threat created by a disorder in the body or outside world that created an imbalance in the bodily elements of air, fire, earth and water. As the factors causing illness were everywhere and were unstable and unpredictable, they 'represented a [continual] source of danger

… villagers lived in a chronic condition of uncertainty concerning their vulnerability' (Coderey, 2015, 269). They 'bracketed out' this uncertainty in a number of ways. Their daily routines included religious rituals that enhanced karma, 'building up a stock of good fortune, enabling them to maintain individuals and societal well-being' (p. 270).

Over the past 200 years, there has been a significant change in patterns of living, with most people, especially in high-income countries, living in small households in societies of strangers. In the UK, there were nearly 28 million households in 2019, with an average size of 2.4. Nearly 30 per cent of these households, 8.2 million, were single adult households (ONS, 2019). Most households have neighbours, but these neighbours do not have an obligation to become involved in intimate matters. Beyond the neighbourhood are strangers, and interactions with strangers are structured around recognised roles and activities; they are grounded in politeness, a way of interacting without aggression (Brown and Levinson, 1987). The limited resources available within each household and from informal sources outside it, means that when faced with challenge of serious illness, individuals have to rely on specialist health services to manage the situation (Giddens, 1991, pp 161–2).

There are also major cultural difference between belief systems and knowledge in intimate societies and modern large-scale societies. In intimate societies, the knowledge that shapes responses to illness such as belief in supernatural powers forms part of the doxa, which Bourdieu (1977) defines as the taken-for-granted and accepted truths that structure experience of the social and natural worlds. In modern societies, such knowledge has increasingly been converted into expert scientific knowledge, such as the medical knowledge that underpins health-care systems. This scientific knowledge is extensive and complex; it has been codified and taught in medical schools and teaching hospitals. Increasingly, the delivery of health care is grounded in codified knowledge, with decisions about treatment based on clinical protocols and agreed and policed rules. There is at any one time a consensus within medical specialisms about the causes and treatment of specific illness. However, this orthodoxy can be challenged both from within or outside the scientific community, an issue discussed in Chapter 8, which considers challenges to the orthodox view of COVID-19.

In intimate societies, seriously ill people were, until the introduction of modern medical facilities, cared for and treated by their kin within the community. In modern societies, individuals can be cared for and treated in their own household, but given the limitation of resources and support, in cases of serious illness they are more likely to be admitted to a hospital so that experts using their specialist technology and knowledge can identify the cause of the illness and provide treatment.

For the patient and their immediate household, serious illness is a major disruption to the normal flow of everyday life. As Giddens has observed, serious illness undermines ontological security, the 'sense of continuity and order in events' (1991, p. 243). Through the process of investigation, diagnosis and treatment, health professionals take on and manage the uncertainty of the illness, converting it into risk, the probability of different outcomes. While doctors acknowledge a range of uncertainties in this process (Fox, 2003), their objective is to contain and manage the patient's uncertainty.

For the ill person, illness is usually an unexpected event; one that removes them from their familiar routine and environment, and transfers them to the unfamiliar setting of the hospital and to the care of strangers. For the patient, the hospital is essentially an abstract system, a setting 'deploying modes of technical knowledge which have validity independent of the practitioner and clients who make use of them' (Giddens, 1991, p. 18). For the doctor, treating patients is part of the routine of their everyday job, and they apply their technical knowledge and skills to the diagnosis and treatment of the illness. While hospitals can be dangerous environments, as Roth (1957) notes, the routines and rituals enable professionals to disregard or bracket out this personal danger.

A way of making sense of and managing uncertainties is time. Timetables provide a way of organising work and of identifying potential risks and managing them. This can be seen in the management of childbirth. As Scamell and Alaszewski (2012) observe, even though childbirth is relatively safe in contemporary society, it is created as a fateful moment, an event where a lot is at stake (p. 208). In their ethnographic study, they found little evidence of a protective cocoon of routine; rather, midwives were aware of the possibility of things going wrong and treated all births as potentially hazardous (p. 213). Midwives managed this uncertainty by following protocols, including the use of a partogram, which charts key parameters such as cervical dilation, fetal heart rate and maternal blood pressure. Such routine surveillance provides midwives with a tool to identify any deviance from the norm (Scamell and Alaszewski, 2012, p. 217). As Scamell and Stewart (2014) observe, 'The partogram represents (among other things) a timetable for dilation of the cervix during labour. Women who fail to keep up with this timetable are shifted from a low- to high-risk category and subjected to additional surveillance and intervention' (p. 84).

The relationships between patients and health-care professionals in hospital is essentially an impersonal technical one. It exists to enable the identification of the cause of the illness and provision of treatment and care. This essential impersonality is masked by the use of conventions of sociability to personalise the relationship. As Tanay and her colleagues found in a study of patient/nurse interactions on a cancer ward, humour and joking were used to personalise the relationship – and 'humour helped patients feel comfortable with the nurse' (Tanay et al, 2013).

This personalisation underpins and is expressed in the development of a trusting relationship between patients and those caring for them. Dibben and Lean (2003) examined the strategies that doctors meeting patients for the first time used to rapidly develop and maintain trust. They noted that doctors did not restrict the consultation to the illness; indeed, some parts of the conversation did not 'appear to be concerned with the specific illness in question but, more commonly, revolve around general topics almost wholly unrelated to medical matters' (2003, p. 248). The doctors sought to gain the patient's confidence and cooperation 'to engender compliance [with treatment] through the achievement of a positive sense of patient empowerment' (Dibben and Lean, 2003, p. 253).

Comment

Serious illness disrupts everyday life and threatens its very continuation. In intimate societies, such disruption tends to spread through the whole community, which is mobilised to identify and address the causes, often supernatural, of the danger. In large-scale societies with well-developed health-care systems, serious illness is equally disruptive, but as illness is treated primarily as a private matter, this disruption is contained where possible within individual households, and where this is not possible within the health-care system. Experts use scientific knowledge about the causes of illness, enabling the uncertainty about past (causes of illness), present (diagnoses and treatments) and future (recovery) to be converted into risk, based on probabilities.

When managing their everyday workload, health professionals are engaged in what Horlick-Jones refers to as risk work. There are uncertainties and ambiguities, but risk work involves making sense of these ambiguities and taking 'risk-related action in ways that not only make sense, but also present them in a "good" or morally acceptable light'(Horlick-Jones, 2005, p. 298). Thus, risk work involves identifying risks, taking action to mitigate them and accounting for those actions.

Hospitals, professional staff and the pandemic

During the COVID-19 pandemic, there was a major shift in the nature and management of serious illness, and a reversal of the normal accepted relationship between the public and the health-care system. In normal times, the public are invited to treat hospitals as safe places where they will be protected, cared for and treated. During the COVID-19 pandemic, especially when there was uncontrolled transmission of the virus in the community, hospitals were no longer safe places. The public were asked to protect the hospitals; for example, in the UK, the government slogan included the phrase

'PROTECT THE NHS'. Patients admitted to hospital and staff working in them were in danger of contracting COVID-19. Access to hospital and other health-care facilities was restricted and all non-essential services ceased.

The impact of governments' requests to minimise use of health care can be seen in data from the US and UK. In the US, the CDC found that attendance at emergency departments across the US dropped by 42 per cent in the first wave of the pandemic, from 2.1 million per week in early April 2019 to 1.2 million in the same period in 2020 (CDC, 2020c). In England, there was a similar drop: in April to June 2019, there were 6,392,158 attendances, while from April to June 2020, there were 3,589,729 attendances (NHS, 2021). As Rachel Clarke noted when she was shown round the Emergency Department of John Radcliffe Hospital (a prestigious teaching hospital in Oxford) at the start of the first wave: 'today ... the typical soundtrack of a city ED [Emergency Department]—are replaced by an uncanny quiet ... the patients we would usually expect in the ED have vanished electing not to come. ... The government's messaging is actively urging such stoicism. Stay at home, we're told repeatedly. Protect the NHS' (Clarke, 2021, pp 118–19).

The reduction in services had a major impact on the treatment of non-COVID-19 patients. After a year of the pandemic, more than 4.5 million people in the UK were waiting to start treatment and 225,000 had been waiting over a year for admission to hospital (Gallagher, 2021). The number of heart operations had fallen from 473,000 in 2019 to 371,000 in 2020, and there were 5,700 excess deaths from heart conditions and strokes in England.

The overwhelming of hospitals

The pandemic changed the nature, experience and risks of illness. At the start of the pandemic, it was possible to trace the path of the virus as it moved between countries, overwhelming their hospitals and necessitating crisis action both inside hospitals (reprovisioning) and outside (lockdowns) to protect them.

On 24 January 2020, Fifield (2020) reported on the impact of the virus on hospitals in Wuhan, the epicentre of the first outbreak. His article drew on videos and commentary posted on social media to provide a picture of what was happening. The videos showed that the hospitals were experiencing extreme levels of stress. Online posts from staff confirmed this. For example, a nurse working in Xincheng Hospital posted a message on WeChat, a messaging app, saying that 'The situation out here is grim. ... All major hospitals in Wuhan are full to the brim and have run out of space. There is simply no room to admit any more cases' (Fifield, 2020).

The impact of the pandemic was clear in a fly-on-the-wall documentary recorded in four Wuhan hospitals in early February 2020; it was broadcast in the US and UK in 2021. The documentary opens with a distressing scene of four people dressed in full PPE running along a hospital corridor and then stopping at a ward door. It becomes clear that one of the four is a women whose father is in the ward, and the others are preventing her from entering as he is dying of COVID-19. There follows a scene in which staff in full PPE are clearly struggling to learn how to use equipment, and one nurse comments that they are full and can take no more patients. There are patients banging on the door to be admitted (YouTube, 2020c).

The first signs that SARS-CoV-2 had reached Europe and was spreading uncontrollably in the community came from Italy in late February 2020. Hospitals in Lombardy in the north of the country had a sudden surge of COVID-19 cases and rapidly ran out of beds, especially beds with ventilators in ICU. On 12 March, the region had 737 ICU beds of which 600 were full, and demand was rising (Harlan and Pitrelli, 2020). The region had 4,200 COVID-19 patients, and the head of Lombardy's ICU anticipated that within two weeks this would rise to 20,000, with up to 4,000 needing ICU treatment. Indeed, as the pressure of admissions increased, so staff concerns started to shift from the safety of the patients to their own safety (Harlan and Pitrelli, 2020).

In the UK, London was the first city to be hit by the pandemic. In early February 2020, Public Health England asked Northwick Park Hospital in London to prepare to screen incoming passengers from Wuhan (Mackintosh, 2020). Given this warning, staff in the hospital engaged in rigorous training for the anticipated influx of patients. On 3 March, they admitted their first suspect patient, a passenger from Iran, who was followed rapidly by two further confirmed cases. By 8 March, managers and senior staff had decided to divide the hospital into two parts, one for non-COVID-19 patients and the other for COVID-19 patients. There followed a rapid increase in COVID-19 admissions, and they opened two new wards for COVID-19 patients on 9 March; within two days, these were full. Cases were doubling every two days (Mackintosh, 2020). By 19 March, numbers had risen so far that the hospital was being overwhelmed. It declared an emergency, and all new cases were diverted to other hospitals. Dr Rachel Tennant, one of the specialists dealing with COVID-19 patients, described the situation: 'We knew Covid was coming. … It had been in the news since January and we were preparing around February. Then it hit us like a tonne of bricks. It hit us hard and fast – the epicentre of the outbreak in the UK' (Mackintosh, 2020).

The pandemic hit New York at about the same time. At Wyckoff Heights Medical Center in Brooklyn, the first COVID-19 patient was admitted on 4 March; she died on 14 March, the first confirmed COVID-19 death in New York (Shuster, 2020). Unlike Northwick Park, Wyckoff Heights had made little preparation for COVID-19: there was only one room in intensive care that could manage highly infectious patients. As the numbers rose, it became difficult to sustain staff numbers: of the 1,800 full-time staff, approximately 25 per cent were absent at some time during the first wave. As a result, the remaining staff had to work long shifts, caring for three times as many patients as normal. At the end of March, the Governor of New York issued a plea to other states to support and take patients from New York. In April, the American military deployed a hospital ship, USNS *Comfort*, which took COVID-19 patients from New York hospitals (Shuster, 2020).

Responding to the pressure on hospitals

Hospitals took measures to protect themselves and their staff and to continue functioning in the pandemic. They shut down non-essential services, using the space and staff for the treatment of COVID-19 patients, and internally reorganised. In his autobiographical account of the pandemic in Edinburgh, Gavin Francis, a general practitioner, described the reduction of non-essential medical services as follows:

> [In mid-April] We GPs were sent a message of praise from the hospital, thanking us for doing so well at keeping people away. But it was becoming more difficult to field patient frustration at the shutting down of much of what the NHS used to do: no outpatient clinics, no colonoscopies, no IVF, no ultrasound scans. Even cancer services had been stripped back to essentials, and many routine lab tests had been cancelled to create capacity for coronavirus testing. (Francis, 2021, pp 89–90)

The internal reorganisations involved creating safe non-COVID-19 areas alongside areas for the reception and treatment of patients who had or were likely to have COVID-19. Rachel Clarke recorded these changes 'The first patients with coronavirus arrived in Oxford's John Radcliffe Hospital in February ... by the first week of March, the entire first floor of the hospital had been dissected into red [COVID-19] and blue [non-COVID-19] zones' (Clarke, 2021, p. 108).

In the Netherlands, de Graaff and his colleagues (2021) monitored the changes in a teaching hospital as COVID-19 admissions rose rapidly in March 2020. Using data from an organisational ethnography, they identified different elements of risk work. At strategic level, the hospital initiated crisis meetings of all key decision makers (managers and senior clinicians). At the peak of the first wave, these were daily, but became less frequent as the lockdown eased pressure on the hospital. These meetings tended to focus on numbers and stocktaking:

> Counting the (lack of) available IC-beds was the very first thing participants in these crisis meetings did in response to the dashboard-like

situation report provided to them detailing even more numbers to be worked with and discussed – ranging from stock-levels of PPE to outflow of recovered COVID-19 patients to long-term care facilities… (de Graaff, Bal and Bal, 2021, p. 116)

This balancing of demand for resources, especially the number of COVID-19 patients and the seriousness of their illness, and the supply of resources, including ICU beds, staff and PPE, was a key element in the risk work that enabled the hospital to remain open.

Alongside the risk work on numbers, de Graaff and his colleagues identified risk work relating to medical expertise. This took place in an Outbreak Management Team, which was chaired by a micro-biologist and brought together clinicians from a range of departments. These experts addressed the practical problems of controlling the spread of the virus within the hospital and keeping services working. For example, they identified as a main risk 'the probabilities hospital staff faced [of] becoming infected while delivering care and, in turn, infecting other staff and patients. But that had to be weighed against another risk – that of running out of PPE' (de Graaff, Bal and Bal, 2021, p. 119). They also considered the risk of allowing patients to have visitors, balancing 'risks of infection for staff, scarce PPE without which care would halt, and the appreciation of family in need of visiting their (dying) relatives' (de Graaff, Bal and Bal, 2021, p. 119).

In normal times such risks tend to be managed through protocols – nationally agreed, evidenced-based written procedures. However, during the pandemic, existing protocols were no longer relevant, so experts in the hospital (microbiologists and clinicians) created new ones that drew on their tacit knowledge, the expertise that they had developed through practice and on the 'deluge of COVID-19 research' (de Graaff, Bal and Bal, 2021, p. 119) in other hospitals and research centres. They often accessed such research through informal channels such as app groups and (evening) video calls. This risk work also drew on studies within the hospital, for example 'to analyse if and which PPE would be reusable, or to determine which operations posed a higher risk … through the release of aerosols, and thus would need a higher quality of PPE' (de Graaff, Bal and Bal, 2021, p. 119).

There was a third element of risk work: regional and supra-regional co-ordination. Hospitals in the Netherlands did not work in isolation: if one was in danger of being overwhelmed and might be forced to triage patients to protect scare ICU resources, then it could reduce the pressure by transferring patients to other hospitals – even ones in Germany. However, such cooperation was sensitive, as senior staff in hospitals had pride and honour and were unwilling to admit their hospital could not cope. The logistics of moving patients to hospitals that had spare capacity therefore required sensitive negotiations, and this was undertaken by a national centre for allocating patients. This negotiated with hospitals to ensure that they had up-to-date information about bed availability and demand, and between 21 March and 10 April 2020, about 770 patients were transferred between hospitals (de Graaff, Bal and Bal, 2021, p. 122).

Fear and anxiety among health-care staff

In health-care systems, there are protocols for ensuring risk are safely managed, and in normal times, health workers are willing to accept these risks. However, the pandemic changed the nature of those risks. The disruption of the health-care system and of normal daily routines and activities, as well as a lack of knowledge about the new virus, created a sense of fear. Doctors and other staff who were normally protected. were in danger of contracting the virus. Media, especially social media, coverage of pandemic highlighted the danger to health professionals. The case of Li Wenliang, an ophthalmologist in Wuhan, was widely reported. On 31 December 2019, Li posted a warning to his colleagues on social media about COVID-19 cases in his hospital. He then contracted the virus and was admitted to hospital on 12 January. While in hospital, he posted an image of himself seriously ill with COVID-19. He died on 7 February (Clarke, 2021, pp. 36–8).

In a small longitudinal study of health professionals during the first COVID-19 wave in the Netherlands, van der Molen and Brown (2021) examined the ways in which the virus disrupted the routines of hospital work, creating new uncertainties and the ways in which professionals sought to make sense of and protect themselves. At the start of the first wave, health professionals in the study were alerted to the new disease by social and mass media reporting. Van der Molen and Brown (2021) observed that the participants in their study became aware of the new virus through media coverage, such as the overwhelming of hospitals in northern Italy. The threat of this new virus undermined participants' sense of personal ontological security and their ability to bracket out risk to themselves. They were aware that their hospital could be overwhelmed, and were concerned whether their hospital had sufficient staff and resources to cope with the coming wave of admissions (van der Molen and Brown, 2021, p. 459). They were also anxious about their own personal safety and the 'risk to the self through infection' (van der Molen and Brown, 2021, p. 459). The participants were aware that they could protect themselves using PPE, but were uncertain about its availability, use and maintenance. When the first wave arrived, services were not overwhelmed and, despite shortages of PPE, staff were able to cope, but as the wave waned, so participants started to worry about the next one. Participants used the same strategies that patients use to manage uncertainties about the future: trust and hope, even fatalism.

The pandemic disrupted health and social care services and undermined the routines that enabled health professionals to bracket out risk. Van de Molen and Brown (2021) observed that one way in which the participants in their study coped with the threat of COVID-19 was to establish new routines and rituals. For example, participants described the ways in hospitals developed protocols that established new working practices. In most hospitals, space was divided into 'clean' (uninfected) and 'dirty' (COVID-19-infected) areas with clear boundaries and different working practices. One participant described everyday working protocols:

> on the left side, (you have) the dirty side, and on the righthand side the clean side. On the clean side you put your clothes on. There are the clean things so you didn't touch anything there if you had touched anything with Corona[virus]. … And then on the other [dirty] side you took your suit off. There you had to put your used apron, your surgical mask, so it could all be [cleaned and] reused. (van der Molen and Brown, 2021, p. 464)

As van der Molen and Brown noted, participants felt that such protocols created a 'well-organised' space that minimised the risk of infection, and 'the clarity and consistency of these systematised routines and boundary-making, or rituals, in relation to dirt 'ensured [their] safety' (van der Molen and Brown, 2021, p. 464).

Comment

During the COVID-19 pandemic, especially at the start of the first wave, the new virus changed the normal distribution and experience of risk. In normal times, serious illness disrupts the lives of an ill person and their immediate family and friends, creating danger and uncertainty. In countries with well-developed health-care systems, health-care professionals can minimise and contain this disruption by converting uncertainty into measurable risk and providing hope of treatment and recovery. During the pandemic, the health system and those working in it could no longer contain this disruption and danger; indeed, their own lives were disrupted, and they and their families were in danger.

Case Study 7: PPE and risk

The development of PPE

Laura Spinney (2018) observed that during the 1918–1919 flu pandemic there was no medical consensus about how medical and other staff should protect themselves from infection, but that in some countries they were advised to wear layered gauze masks over their mouths as protection. She noted that in Japan mask wearing was adopted by the general public outside hospitals (Spinney, 2018, p. 97). As Roth argued in his classic study of infection control in a tuberculosis facility, measures to protect against infections such as the wearing of protective equipment are shaped by cultural factors, including perception of the risk of infection. He noted that hospital staff were expected to wear protective clothing (masks, gowns and hair coverings) when they come into contact with patients, but often did not. He observed that staff of the higher rank seemed 'to have the privilege of taking the greater risks, particularly in the case of masks' (Roth, 1957, p. 312). The routines of everyday activities tended to bracket out the threat of infection. In the COVID-19 pandemic, the disruption of routines undermined such bracketing out.

As the understanding of the mechanics of viral spread and the technology of protective equipment developed in the 20th century, so the range of equipment available to protect health workers from infection increased. By the beginning of the 21st century, workers could be offered either limited protection from contact or droplet transmission, with protective gloves, plastic aprons and face masks and/or visors, or more comprehensive protection, with complete body covering providing protection from all biohazards.

In the Ebola outbreak, some infected individuals travelled from West Africa to the US. The CDC guidance was that those treating Ebola patients should wear gloves, a gown and a mask or other face covering (CDC, 2007, IV. B). However this protection proved inadequate. When a Liberian man was treated in a Dallas hospital, he vomited and had diarrhoea, and both the nurses treating him contracted Ebola (Mohan, 2014). On 20 October 2014, the CDC updated its guidance. It acknowledged that Ebola could be spread by droplet infection, and stated that those treating Ebola patients should wear PPE that covered their whole body, with no skin or mouth exposure (CDC, 2014).

PPE and COVID-19

At the start of the COVID-19 pandemic, WHO (2020e) issued guidance on the type of protection that health care and others working with COVID-19 patients should have. It indicated that protection should be risk based. In lower risk care settings, WHO recommended basic protection of gloves, gowns and masks, which should be upgraded in higher risk setting with COVID-19 positive and aerosol spray, for example caused by invasive procedures (WHO, 2020e).

CDC guidance for health-care settings in the US was more detailed. It indicated that health-care workers in all facilities should take control measures such as wearing masks to prevent droplet spread and also that all patients and visitors to a facility should do likewise during their stay in the facility (CDC, 2020d). In areas where there was community transmission but health-care workers were not working with COVID-19 patients, they should still take precautions and wear a mask fitted with a respirator (N95 mask) and eye protection. When they were working with patients suspected of or confirmed as having COVID-19, they should wear a mask fitted with a respirator, a clean isolation gown properly tied, gloves and eye protection (CDC, 2021e).

PPE stockpiles

In their contingency planning for a future pandemic, most high-income countries had built up stockpiles of PPE. In the US, the federal government created a Strategic National Stockpile of protective equipment in 1999, enabling rapid response to chemical or nuclear attacks. This was expanded to provide resources to respond to terrorism, hurricanes, H1N1 flu and Ebola (Sherman, 2020). These stockpiles are an insurance against relatively rare events that are by their nature low probability but high consequence. Therefore, when government budgets are under stress, cutting expenditure on stockpiling provides an easy way of making savings.

In a Coronavirus Task Force briefing at the White House on 6 April 2020, President Trump claimed that the US response to COVID-19 had been undermined by the lack of a PPE stockpile, and that at the start of the pandemic:

> they also gave us empty cupboards. The cupboard was bare. You've heard the expression, the cupboard was bare. So we took over a stockpile with a cupboard was bare and where the testing system was broken and old and we redid it and frankly it would be okay for a small event but not for a big event and they had a chance to do it. (Rev, 2020b)

POLITIFACT reviewed the evidence (Sherman, 2020), and concluded that Trump had exaggerated. There was PPE in the stockpile but it had been run down during the Obama administration: in particular, the N95 masks used during the 2009 swine flu (H1N1) epidemic had not been replaced. This meant that while the stockpile was full of equipment, it was 'not enough to handle this particular pandemic. Most notably, the stockpile was short of N95 masks' (Sherman, 2020).

In the UK, the government was confident at the start of the pandemic that its Influenza Preparedness Programme stockpile was adequate. On 17 March 2020, when questioned by the chair of the Select Committee on Health and Social Care, Sir Simon Stevens, the Chief Executive of NHS

England and NHS Improvement, stated: 'as we sit here today, nationally the Department of Health and Social Care procurement team has sufficient for the PPE that we are going to need over the coming weeks, but there is a distributional issue around the country and we are going to need more of it' (Health and Social Care Committee, 2020, Q 131).

This statement turned out to be hopelessly optimistic. As the first wave hit the UK in late March, it rapidly emerged that there was a shortage of key equipment. The Influenza Preparedness Programme was stockpiling equipment for a flu pandemic, but given the differences between SARS-CoV-2 and flu viruses, especially the role of aerosol transmission, SARS-CoV-2 required different kinds of protective equipment. The stockpile did not have enough fluid-repellent gowns and visors (Foster and Neville, 2020).

PPE shortages and changing policy

In early March 2020, the WHO warned of a global shortage of PPE, noting that 'Since the start of the COVID-19 outbreak, prices have surged. Surgical masks have seen a sixfold increase, N95 respirators have trebled and gowns have doubled. Supplies can take months to deliver and market manipulation is widespread, with stocks frequently sold to the highest bidder' (WHO, 2020d).

High-income countries such as the US and UK could outbid lower income countries, but at the start of the pandemic they did not have manufacturing capacity. They depended on manufacturers in East Asia, and these supplies were unreliable. In the US, media reports and congressional inquiries indicated persistent shortages of PPE. In July 2020, a *Washington Post* article outlined continuing shortages:

> the inability to secure PPE is especially frustrating, health–care workers say, because it is their main defence against catching the virus. For weeks, nurses have posted online testimonials about a lack of PPE, with some given surgical masks instead of N95 masks because of shortages. In a video posted last week, a Florida nurse said she breaks the oath she took 'to do no harm' every time she goes to work without protection and worries constantly she may be infecting her patients, co–workers and family. (Wan, 2020)

In the UK, there were similar shortages. Rachel Clarke in her account of the pandemic, describes the shortages as follows:

> Even *after* PPE standards had been downgraded for the majority of frontline staff, the appropriate kit was still unavailable for many of them. Three nurses from the recently overwhelmed Northwick Park

Hospital in London shared a photo of themselves with bin bags on their heads as they issued a plea for proper masks, gowns and gloves. ... Shortly [after the photo], all three nurses tested positive for Covid. (emphasis in the original, Clarke, 2021b)

Health-care staff were aware of media coverage of health workers who did not have access to proper PPE and had contracted COVID-19, becoming seriously ill or even dying. For example, Abdul Mahud Chowdhury, a 53-year-old consultant urologist who worked at Homerton Hospital in east London and had no underlying health problems, died of COVID-19 on 8 April 2020 (Weaver, 2020). Before his death, he had written to Prime Minister Boris Johnson, raising concerns that front-line staff were working in direct contact with COVID-infected patients without access to either testing or PPE (Weaver 2020).

In the first wave of the pandemic, the UK government changed its PPE guidance regularly. At the start of the pandemic, health-care staff treating COVID-19 patients used full PPE, as they had done when treating Ebola patients. On 11 February, the government issued guidance recommending more limited PPE: fluid repellent gowns, gloves, masks with respirators and goggles/visors. In the next two months, the guidance was changed eight times, most notably on 19 March when COVID-19 was reclassified as no longer a high-consequence infectious disease, and therefore 'enhanced' PPE was no longer recommended (Foster and Neville, 2020).

The impact of PPE on health-care staff

The limited supply of PPE and the changing government guidelines undermined health and social care workers' trust in in their employers and in the government. Staff felt that changing guidance did not reflect evidence about the changing virulence of SARS-CoV-2; rather it reflected shortages in the supply of PPE.

The problems over the supply and availability of PPE, reflected an underlying ambiguity and tension over its use. While health and social care staff acknowledged that PPE provided some protection against infection, they also felt it was unpleasant to wear and impeded their ability to care for and communicate with patients.

Health and social care workers noted that wearing PPE interfered in their relationship with patients. It made communication difficult as PPE interfered with both speech and hearing, and it reduced the intimacy that many workers felt was essential for bonding with patients and gaining their trust. In her account of working through the pandemic, Rachel Clarke describes the impact of PPE: 'How hard it is to convey warmth and humanity when trussed up behind a visor and mask. ... But now patients are alone when they long for their loved ones. Everyone they see looks like an alien in a mask' (2021, p. 121).

Risk implications

In normal times, working in health and social care involves some risk, but this is managed as part of routine everyday practice and therefore does not create specific concern and anxiety. The onset of the COVID-19 pandemic changed this: health and social care facilities became the centre of the pandemic, and staff working in them were at risk of contracting COVID-19. PPE provided some protection against this risk, but wearing the equipment was unpleasant and it interfered with normal work activity. Images of facilities with staff all dressed in PPE such as the scenes in the Chinese documentary, '76 Days: Inside Wuhan's Lockdown' (YouTube 2020d), highlighted the existential threat of COVID-19.

Comment

The COVID-19 pandemic has inverted the normal relationship between the health-care system and the rest of society. Normally the health-care system functions to protect individuals and society against the dangers of illness, converting the indeterminate uncertainty of illness into quantifiable risk. Professionals undertake risk work to protect individuals who are at risk. Normally, they bracket out the risk to themselves through the familiar routines of everyday wok practices. The pandemic was an existential threat that undermined both the security of institutions and that of the individuals working in them. Professionals were exposed to and became aware of the risk that the institutions they worked in would be overwhelmed, and that they themselves were at risk. To manage these new uncertainties, professionals developed new knowledge and new routines to provide new certainties and security. However, given the unpredictability of the pandemic, such security was always fragile and professionals often had to rely on default strategies – strategies used when action has to be taken but there is not enough time or knowledge to rationally evaluate alternatives. In-between strategies (Zinn, 2008) such as trust, hope, intuition and fatalism provided ways in which professionals could manage such uncertainty during the pandemic (van der Molen and Brown, 2021).

PART III

Risk narratives

Pandemic narratives: telling stories about COVID-19 and its risks

Pandemic narratives and risk

The media and representations of risk

As Giddens (1999) has observed, a key feature of modernity is the development of new and multiple forms of communication, enabling information to move more rapidly over greater distances. In the 20th century, the well-established print media have been complemented by new modes of communication. Some of these such as televisions and radio broadcasting replicate the structures of the print media. Others such as social media provide new modes that are based on more open access and less scrutiny of the material published.

With the development of different modes of communication, individuals can access information from a range of sources. In modern global societies, events happening in distant places can affect our lives in unexpected ways and we gain knowledge about such events from various media (Giddens, 1999). Such rapid and open communication was evident in the COVID-19 pandemic. The physical spread of the virus was preceded by the spread of information online. On 30 December 2019, the head of the Emergency Department in Wuhan Dental Hospital received a test result carried out by a lab in Beijing marked 'SARS CORONAVIRUS'. She highlighted it in red and passed it to the Chinese messaging site WeChat, which posted it online. This posting was picked up by a local doctor, Li Wenliang, who shared the posting with his university class group, and it rapidly spread. When the local health commission issued orders for local hospitals to report cases to it and not to discuss such cases in public, these orders were leaked online. Dr Marjorie Pollack, deputy editor of ProMed, a programme monitoring the internet for information about disease outbreaks, was alerted to this chatter by a contact in Taiwan. Pollack issued an emergency post on the ProMed network asking for more information, and received notification of a posting on a Chinese business news site confirming early reports. She also received an alert from an artificial intelligence system at Boston's Children Hospital about pneumonia cases in Wuhan. On the basis of this evidence, Pollack issued a warning just before midnight on 31 December 2019, to the ProMed global community, 80,000 doctors, epidemiologists and public health experts, about a new SARS-like disease in Wuhan (McMullen, 2020; Honigsbaum, 2020, pp 261–2).

These multiple channels of communication enable individuals to access representations of the world in addition to those they can obtain directly from their own observations or indirectly from the observations of their friends and family. As Philo and his colleagues (1996) have observed, the mass media play a key role in shaping the representations and understanding of risk. In a study of the media representation of mental illness, they found that individuals gained most of their understanding of its dangers and risk from media representations. When such media representations clashed with their own personal experiences, individuals tended to privilege media representations even if they knew they were fictional, for example in television soap operas.

Pandemics: the development of the narrative matrix as a way of representing risk

While contemporary politicians may claim that the COVID-19 pandemic is unprecedented, there are historical records of similar pandemics. Procopius recorded the impact of the bubonic plague (caused by a bacteria, Yersinia pestis) during the reign of the Byzantine Emperor Justinian I (527–565 CE). The pandemic probably started in China and spread through North India to the Mediterranean, reaching Egypt by 541 and Constantinople around 542, and lasting until 750 CE (Sarris, 2021). In his account of the plague, Procopius described its initial appearance in Egypt and its movement to Constantinople, where he was an eyewitness. He described the signs and symptoms of the disease, noting that it affected individuals in different ways: some experienced delirium and others developed pustules and bled to death. His descriptions of this form of plague are consistent with modern medical descriptions (Procopius, 1914, Book II, 22).

Procopius reflected on the ways in which plague undermined everyday life. He noted that 'At that time all the customary rites of burial were overlooked. For the dead were not carried out escorted by a procession in the customary manner, nor were the usual chants sung over them' (Procopius, 1914, Book II, 23). When existing tombs were filled, bodies were dumped in the city's fortifications. 'As a result of this an evil stench pervaded the city and distressed the inhabitants still more, and especially whenever the wind blew fresh from that quarter' (Procopius, 1914, Book II, 23).

Where Procopius's account of the plague differs from modern accounts is in his analysis of its causes. He observed that the infections and deaths were random and arbitrary, concluding that it was divine retribution for human sins, especially those of the emperor: 'But for this calamity it is quite impossible either to express in words or to conceive in thought any explanation, except indeed to refer it to God' (Procopius, 1914, Book II, 22).

In more recent accounts of epidemics, Procopius's attribution of such disasters to divine wrath is replaced by their treatment as public catastrophes, stemming from a failure to effectively identify and mitigate risk. As Mairal (2011) notes, this shift underpins the development of modern journalism in the 18th century, and was evident in Daniel Defoe's account of the 1665 Plague of London, published in 1722.

Defoe's account of the 1665 Plague was a fictional 'eyewitness' narrative. Defoe created a narrative matrix (Mairal, 2011), combining a subjective and emotional eyewitness account with objective factual evidence, especially the numbers dying each week as recorded in the parish burial records. In the second week of June, Defoe's fictional eyewitness made the following observations: 'at the other End of the Town their Consternation was very great; and the richer sort of People, especially the Nobility and Gentry from the West-part of the City, throng'd out of Town with their Families and Servants in an unusual Manner' (1722, p. 8). Defoe's fictional eyewitness commented on his feelings about the events he was observing and recording.

Albert Camus (1960), in his fictional account of an outbreak of bubonic plague in 1940s Oran, Algeria, used Defoe's narrative matrix. His fictional account drew on 'eyewitnesses' and documents, and combined factual observation with personal reflection. His main protagonist, Dr Bernaud Rieux, a medical doctor, started his account with a description of the sinister warning of the outbreak: dying rats. Rieux documented his exhausting workload alongside his sense of frustration at the slow response of civil authorities and his own powerlessness. He described the ways in which some of his actions, such as removing infected individuals from their houses and families, increased suffering. Camus reflected on the personal experience of lockdown, including the strange combination of boredom and fear (Camus, 1960, p. 173).

Within a year of the start of the COVID-19 pandemic, there were already a number of published narratives based on the pandemic. These were often written by doctors: accounts by Gavin Francis (2021), a GP, and Rachel Clarke (2021), a palliative care doctor, are examples. Clarke used the same device as Defoe and Camus to tell her story, an eyewitness account: 'I needed, I think, to take a stand with my pen and simply say: I was there. I have seen it, from the inside. I know what it was like. Here, with all its flaws and its inherent subjectivity, is my testimony. Make of it what you will' (2021, p. 18). Having provided a scientific (2021, pp 51–4) and factual context for the COVID-19 pandemic, she recorded the warning signs of the approaching virus and the exponential growth of cases in Lombardy: 'But I am worried. I'm worried sick. By the end of the month [February] there may be only 23 documented cases of the virus in Britain, yet the death toll in Italy is hurtling upwards' (2021, p. 50). The key focus of Clarke's narrative is on the suffering of those dying from the virus, and of their families and those caring for them. Her narrative opened with the description of a man dying:

He lies on the hospital sheets, but he's drowning.

Behind closed doors, with neither fanfare nor drama, he's been quietly drowning all night. The act of voicing distress – altering another human being to his plight – takes spare air he no longer possesses. ... And though the oxygen roars, the highest flow we can manage, it's still not enough, not remotely. (Clarke, 2021, p. 1)

All narratives or stories are told or written for a purpose. Procopius saw the plague as divine retribution for human sinning. Defoe wrote his fictional account to warn Londoners of the dangers of another plague. Camus's plague narrative was a warning of the depersonalisation and dehumanisation of crises, which could be countered by common decency: people helping and looking after each other. In her narrative, Clarke made judgements about how different participants responded to the first four months of the pandemic. She made positive comments about the forbearance of patients and their families, and about the resilience of the NHS and its staff. She was critical of political leaders such as Boris Johnson and Matt Hancock, indicating that they had failed to provide leadership, heed warnings and communicate honestly. She commented: 'How incredulous we have been to see government figures breaking the rules they wrote, that so many others have lived and died by' (Clarke, 2021, p. 215).

Different accounts of the COVID-19 pandemic

The ways in which stories are structured and the devices used reflect the aims of the storyteller, the messages they are trying to communicate. The elements of the narrative matrix evident in Defoe's account are therefore evident in many of the stories told and written about the pandemic and its risks and misfortunes, but the precise elements and their relative balance vary. Representatives of governments aim to warn their populations about the dangers of the virus and the actions that they should take to protect themselves. To establish their credibility and trustworthiness, these representatives tend to emphasise the facts, often represented by numbers, although they may also seek to empathise with the population and the suffering of individuals. Governments, especially in democratic countries, have provided regular accounts of pandemics. The traditional broadcasting media draw on government accounts, but they also have access to other representations of the pandemic, such as those of dissenting scientists, survivors of the virus or friends and relatives of victims. Combining these sources enables the creation of a narrative matrix. Thus, within the broadcast media, such personal accounts feature more prominently, and the voices of victims and those who dissent from the official narrative can be found.

Official accounts: emphasising numbers and facts

On 11 March 2020, the Director General of the WHO, Tedros Ghebreyesus, declared that COVID-19 was a global pandemic. He highlighted the risk of the new virus, stating that 'We [the WHO] have rung the alarm bell loud and clear' (Ghebreyesus, 2020a). He used various facts represented by numbers to highlight the increasing threat of COVID-19:

In the past two weeks, the number of cases of COVID-19 outside China has increased 13-fold, and the number of affected countries has tripled. There are now more than 118,000 cases in 114 countries, and 4,291 people have lost their lives. Thousands more are fighting for their lives in hospitals. (Ghebreyesus, 2020a)

Donald Trump, however, sought to minimise the danger of the new virus, and created a positive narrative in which he was protecting the American population. In his State of the Union Address on 4 February 2020, he stated that the US was working with the Chinese government, and that 'My administration will take all necessary steps to safeguard our citizens from this threat' (*New York Times*, 2020). In his press briefing on 26 February, Trump responded to evidence of community transmission in New York and California and to panic on the stock market by stressing the small numbers of confirmed cases and their good outcome.

As most of you know, the – the level that we've had in our country is very low, and those people are getting better, or we think that in almost all cases they're better, or getting. We have a total of 15. We took in some from Japan. … It [the total number of COVID cases] could have been as many as 42. … Of the 15 people – the 'original 15,' as I call them – 8 of them have returned to their homes, to stay in their homes until fully recovered. One is in the hospital and five have fully recovered. And one is, we think, in pretty good shape and it's in between hospital and going home. (The White House, 2020a)

The aim of Trump's narrative was to reassure the American public that everything was under control and the risks were minimal. When infections and deaths started rising rapidly in March 2020, this narrative was difficult to sustain, so he shifted to an alternative one in which he acknowledged rising deaths but emphasised how many lives his actions had saved:

you're talking about a potential of up to 2.2 million [deaths]. And some people said it could even be higher than that. … And so, if we can hold that down, as we're saying, to 100,000 – that's a horrible

number – maybe even less, but to 100,000; so we have between 100-
and 200,000 – we all, together, have done a very good job. (The
White House, 2020b)

In the UK, the government also tried to control the COVID-19 pandemic
narrative through regular televised briefings, especially during the first wave.
One such was held on 15 April 2020. It had all the key elements of the
narrative matrix: there were scientists (Chris Whitty and Angela McClean,
Deputy CSA) outlining the science and highlighting the key facts, and
Matt Hancock, the Secretary of State, talking about the facts, the shared
national sacrifice, his personal and emotional responses, and the action the
government was taking to protect social care.

Near the start of his presentation, Matt Hancock highlighted key
facts: 'On the most recent figures, 313,769 people have now been tested
for coronavirus. Of these, 98,476 people have tested positive. The number
of patients in hospital with symptoms is now 19,529. 12,868 people have
sadly died, an increase of 761' (Hancock, 2020b). He emphasised that the
virus was dangerous and that the national 'shared sacrifice … is starting to
work' (Hancock 2020b).

In his presentation, Hancock talked about two individuals, Captain
Tom Moore and Ismail Mohamed Abdulwahab. Captain Tom Moore was
an elderly care home resident who was to raise over £32 million for the
NHS and receive a knighthood in July 2020 for his efforts (Penna, 2020).
Hancock said: 'I want to pay a special tribute today to Captain Tom Moore
who, at the age of 99, has raised over £7 million so far for NHS charities
by completing 100 laps of his garden. Captain Tom, you're an inspiration
to us all and we thank you' (Hancock, 2020b).

Hancock then went on to talk about one of the innocent victims, Ismail
Abdulwahab, a 13-year-old boy who had died on 30 March. His family was
unable to attend his funeral as two of his siblings showed signs of COVID-19.
Matt Hancock talked about his emotional response to Ismail's death: 'As a father
of a 13-year-old myself, the reports of Ismail, dying aged 13 without a parent
at his bedside, made me weep. And the sight of his coffin being lowered into a
grave without a member of his family present was too awful' (Hancock, 2020b).

The key message of the briefing came next. The government was being
criticised for its failure to protect front-line staff by not providing PPE and
for failing to protect the residents of care homes by allowing the discharge
of untested patients from hospitals to care homes. He stated that the PPE
plan announced on 9 April would be extended to include social care staff.
He noted the government had injected an extra £1.6 billion into social
care, and announced that the government priority was to control the spread
of infection in social care and ensure care home residents discharged from
hospital were tested (Hancock, 2020b).

As the pandemic progressed, so the Downing Street briefings became more irregular. When the prime minister announced the move from Plan A to Plan B on 12 December 2021, in response to the new Omicron variant, it took the form of a pre-recorded Address to the Nation with no supporting scientists or questions from the press. There was a factual element in Johnson's statement. He reported: 'Earlier today, the UK's four CMOs raised the Covid Alert level to 4, its second highest level, because of the evidence that Omicron is doubling here in the UK every two to three days' (Johnson, 2021e). He then made a risk assessment based on past evidence: 'We know from bitter experience how these exponential curves develop. No-one should be in any doubt: there is a tidal wave of Omicron coming' (Johnson, 2021e). He added: 'Do not make the mistake of thinking Omicron can't hurt you; can't make you and your loved ones seriously ill' (Johnson, 2021e), and noted that the coming wave of Omicron 'would risk a level of hospitalisation that could overwhelm our NHS and lead sadly to very many deaths' (Johnson, 2021e).

The prime minister then outlined the ways in which the government proposed to mitigate the risk. The main response was a roll-out of a third or booster jab of COVID-19 vaccine (Johnson, 2021e). Alongside this, he announced measures designed to reduce transmission, including a requirement to wear face masks in indoor public spaces, working from home if possible and, subject to parliamentary approval, restrictions on access to nightclubs and large events.

Johnson's statement was brief and technical with few personal or emotional elements, apart from a reference to 'our wall of vaccine protection to keep our friends and loved ones safe' (Johnson 2021e).

Media narratives: adding moral judgements and emotion to numbers and facts

Broadcast media used governments as a major source of information when reporting figures and narratives. However, they also accessed information from other sources, including those who were directly affected by the pandemic.

Using personal narratives to highlight personal sacrifices and suffering

In the US, ABC News broadcast and posted regular reports on those who had died during the pandemic. At the start of the pandemic, the broadcaster posted a report included the photos, names, ages and occupations of those who had died. The commentary stated 'We want to highlight some of the people who have lost their lives to this pandemic. They are more than statistics' (Shapiro et al, 2020). By 26 December 2020, the commentary and posting had increased, with a commentary for each person plus a Facebook, Twitter or Instagram obituary that often included a photo. The introductory commentary noted that the disease had affected all age groups and individuals from all walks of life, including 'first responders and medical staff – who have been working so diligently and selflessly to stem the tide of the infection and care for the sick' (Shapiro et al, 2020).

In the case of front-line workers, the postings usually included comments on their heroic devotion to duty during the pandemic. The posting for Mohammed Jawed, a 59-year-old small town Kentucky doctor who died on 31 October 2020 reported that he had been diagnosed with myeloma but had returned to practice six months before his death. His eldest daughter said: 'He wanted to continue helping his patients. ... He didn't want to drop the ball on anyone' (Shapiro et al, 2020). The tweet accompanying the posting indicated that the Kentucky state governor had declared Mohammed a hero for sticking with his patients during the pandemic.

The individual postings often highlighted the speed with which the virus killed and the shock and grief of family and workmates. The posting for Lizzy Torres Sanchez, a 31-year-old mother of two, who died on 31 July 2020, recorded that she was six months pregnant and she died several days after her baby died. Her brother-in-law described the response of her family: 'I've never, ever seen so much grief and sadness as I've seen with this. ... A few days before she got sick, she was here at the house and we were talking about life and what she was going to name her baby' (Shapiro et al, 2020).

Heroic stories: overcoming the odds

In the UK, the broadcast media also highlighted stories that illustrated the impact the pandemic was having on individuals. Some of these stories reflected the 'heroic' responses to the pandemic, such as the Captain Tom story.

Media coverage of Tom Moore's charity walking grew rapidly in April 2020. On 15 April, *The Sun* newspaper (Pietras and Sims, 2020) published an update on his walk, reporting that he had raised £7 million. The online version of the article included videos and photos, with a 1940 photo of Tom in his officer's uniform.

Unlike many media reports, Captain Tom's story did not have a short or limited shelf-life. Indeed, it developed over the pandemic and he became a media celebrity. For example, in October 2020, Grant Shapps, the Secretary of State for Transport launched the veterans' railcard scheme, presenting the first railcard to Captain Tom (Starkey, 2020). When Captain Tom died from COVID-19 on 2 February 2021, he received a hero's funeral: his funeral coffin was carried by soldiers and there was a gun salute. The event was covered by national and international media (Patil, 2021).

Captain Tom's story had both an emotional and moral dimension. Emotionally, it was a heart-warming, feel-good story of an elderly man overcoming his limited mobility to raise a substantial amount of money for a good cause. Morally, it fell in the heroic category of personal triumph over COVID-19, albeit with a twist at the end.

Highlighting emotional and moral issues

In the UK, *The Guardian* newspaper regularly published articles featuring accounts of specific individuals who had died during the pandemic. These stories reflected the changing nature of the pandemic. In October 2020, *The Guardian* published an article highlighting the continued impact of the virus during the summer when there were no restrictions on social activities and the government was encouraging economic and social activity. Using official statistics, Mohdin (2020) showed that between 15 June and 8 September 2020, 3,173 people had died. Mohdin focused on the deaths of six individuals, highlighting the ways in which their deaths represented a loss to the community. For example. she wrote about the death of Wilbald Tesha, a mental health nurse who had migrated from Tanzania to work in the NHS. Mohdin included a quote from one of Tesha's former patients, Samantha Chung: 'He was compassionate, understanding, and non-judgmental. He always said hello with a big smile. He was full of positivity and hope for all of us patients. ... I really do owe him my life' (Mohdin, 2020).

Towards the end of 2021, *The Guardian* published a series of stories under the heading 'Lost to the Virus'. These were individual case studies, 'the stories of people who died of Covid-19 – and the systemic failure that may have contributed [to their deaths]' (*The Guardian*, 2021). The article published on 23 November 2021 (Kale, 2021) was an extensive account of the life and death of Samantha Willis, 'a beloved young pregnant woman', who had decided to delay her COVID-19 vaccination until after the birth of her baby, and died two weeks after her baby was born. In the article, her husband, Josh, explained why she delayed being vaccinated:

> Samantha's illness and death was unexpected. She was only 35 and in good health, with no underlying conditions. Samantha was unvaccinated – she had received advice against getting jabbed at an antenatal appointment. 'They gave her a flyer telling her there wasn't enough research on the Covid vaccine in pregnant women,' says Josh. He found the flyer among her things recently. It read: 'The vaccines have not yet been tested in pregnancy, so until more information is available, those who are pregnant should not routinely have this vaccine.' (Kale, 2021)

The article explored the shock and grief of her family. Her husband noted that they had been careful – 'We thought we'd be safe in the house' – and even when they tested positive for COVID-19, they thought that it would be a mild illness: 'It didn't even cross our minds that we would get sick' (Kale, 2021). He said: 'I wish I had done a lot more for her. ... I thought we had another 50 years or so, to watch the wee ones grow up' (Kale, 2021).

The article examined who was responsible for this advice. Kale interviewed Stella Creasy, an MP who had been pregnant at the same time as Samantha and had received the same advice. Creasy stated that she had raised the matter with the minister responsible for vaccines, Nadine Zahawi, and Anthony Harden representing the JCVI. Despite emerging evidence that pregnant women and their unborn foetuses were at risk from COVID-19, they 'kept saying to me that a pregnant woman is at no greater risk of dying than her non-pregnant counterpart' (Kale, 2021). The article blamed male policy makers for the failure to protect pregnant women. Joeli Brearley, the founder of the maternity campaign group, Pregnant Then Screwed, observed: 'If you look at who was on the Covid war cabinet and leading the daily briefing, it was nearly all men. ... Pregnant women ... were just not a priority' (Kale 2021). Brearley indicated that this was 'part of a pattern of generalised apathy towards pregnant women from policymakers' (Kale, 2021).

Journalists used official sources and statistics to identify social groups that have experienced disproportionate levels of infections and deaths. They also used personal stories to illustrate the emotions, such as sadness and loss, and moral implications, especially the injustice of such illnesses and deaths.

Case Study 8: Telling the story of the failure to protect vulnerable residents in care homes in a TV documentary

The failure to protect residents (and staff) in care homes was evident in a number of high-income countries. A *Washington Post* article cited evidence that in 26 such countries 'elder-care home residents have accounted for an average of 47 percent of recorded coronavirus deaths' (Taylor, 2020).

In the UK, a BBC *Panorama* documentary on deaths in care homes was broadcast on 30 July 2020 (BBC 2020b). The documentary noted that at the time of transmission, 22,000 care home residents in the UK had died following a COVID-19 diagnosis (BBC, 2020b). The documentary focused on the experiences of staff and residents in two care homes, one in the north and the other in the south of England.

Alison Holt, the reporter, said that in late February, as evidence emerged of community transmission in Italy, Spain and Austria, the official advice in the UK was that transmission in care homes was unlikely and they should continue operating as usual. Mark Adams the head of a charity, Community Integrated Care, that managed one of the care homes that featured in the documentary, commented: 'In early March, we were seeing what was happening in Italy and Spain and parts of America which was terrifying, including care homes where many people died in outbreaks [of COVID-19]. The writing was on the wall' (BBC, 2020b).

Adams recalled how in the absence of any guidance from government, his charity set up its own 'war room', which identified the main risks their residents faced, and took measures to mitigate these risks. When, on 13 March 2020, the government changed its guidance, advising care homes to only allow in those who were COVID-19-free, the charity decided to lock down all its homes, stopping all visiting. However, within days the virus had been introduced into their Lancashire care home. Dorothy Kierney, one of the residents, had been admitted to hospital with breathing difficulties and was discharged to the home despite having tested positive for COVID-19. She was cared for in isolation by staff wearing protective equipment. She died three days after her return, and the virus spread rapidly through the home. Commenting on the rapid deterioration of two of the residents, a nurse commented that 'it was so frustrating that we were unable to see or predict this'. The home did not have access to COVID-19 tests. The documentary recorded the death of another of the residents, Joan Day. She was lively and active when she was admitted a few months earlier, but when she contracted COVID-19, she rapidly deteriorated. The documentary showed the duty nurse administering morphine to relieve Joan's pain. Joan died later in the day, and the nurse who had taken over Joan's care, who was also caring for five other residents with COVID-19, phoned Joan's daughter, Michelle, to give her the bad news. Michelle said: 'It's the worst feeling in the world.'

The *Panorama* programme told the care home story by highlighting the suffering and emotional responses of staff, residents and their families. It also allocated responsibility for the failure to protect the vulnerable residents. The programme argued that during the early stages of the pandemic the government had prioritised protecting the NHS to ensure that there were sufficient hospital beds. Social care was 'an afterthought'.

Case Study 9: BAMEs and narratives of innocent victims and the guilty parties

The media has highlighted the impact of COVID-19 on a number of vulnerable groups, but one group in particular has attracted attention, individuals from ethnic minority backgrounds. As epidemiologists collected data in the US and the UK, it became clear that the pandemic was affecting some ethnic groups more than others. In October 2020 in the US, individuals with Asian (40 deaths per 100,000 people) or White (47 per 100,000) backgrounds had the lowest death rates, while individuals from other ethnic backgrounds had higher rates: Latinos (65 per 100,000), Pacific Islanders (72 per 100,000), Indigenous Americans (82 per 100,000) and Black Americans (96 per 100,000) (Scott and Animashuan, 2020).

In the UK, the difference was even more marked. The Health Foundation, an independent UK charity, used data published by the Office of National Statistics (2 March–10 April 2020) to explore the relative risks of ethnic groups in England and Wales. Elwell-Sutton, Deeny and Stafford (2020) found that all non-White ethnic groups had an increased relative risk over people of White ethnicity. When controlled for age, individuals of mixed ethnicity and Chinese ethnicity, it nearly doubled; for those with an Indian ethnicity it was nearly two and half times higher and for those from a Black ethnic background it was over four times as high. Adjusting for risk factors such as prior medical conditions, Elwell-Sutton, Deeny and Stafford (2020) found that 'black and Asian people still had around double the risk of dying from COVID-19'.

Awareness of the vulnerability of individuals from ethnic minority backgrounds developed in the early stages of the pandemic as the majority of the early deaths among front-line workers in the UK were from this group. For example, in April 2020, Mary Agyapong was the first reported COVID-19 death of a pregnant women in the UK. Both the tabloid press (Crowson and Bennett, 2020) and broadsheets covered the story, attributing her premature death to the failure of the government to provide her and other pregnant front-line health workers with adequate protection.

The media coverage of the impact of COVID-19 on the BAME community in the US

The pandemic occurred in a highly political environment. On 25 May 2020, a White police officer in Minneapolis was filmed kneeling on the neck of and killing George Floyd, a 46-year-old Black man (Woodward, 2020a, p. 236). There was a major wave of protests in the US asserting that 'Black Lives Matter'. Most of these were peaceful and short lived, though in some cities, such as Portland in Oregon, they were both longer lasting and violent, involving clashes between Black Lives Matter supporters and White supremacist groups such as the Proud Boys (Shen, 2020). In the first presidential debate, Joe Biden, the Democratic candidate, attacked Donald Trump for failing to protect ethnic minorities: 'This is a president who has used everything as a dog whistle to try to generate racist hatred, racist division. This is a man who in fact, he talks about helping African Americans, one in 1000 African Americans has been killed because of the coronavirus' (USA Today, 2020).

In the US, there was media coverage of the impact of COVID-19 on Black Americans. The Washington Post carried an article co-written by two Black female psychiatrists reflecting on their experience of providing support for

Black women during the pandemic. They started with the observation by the former first lady, Michelle Obama, that she was 'experiencing "low-grade depression" caused by the double pandemic of COVID-19 and racial strife' (Jackson and Pederson, 2020). They noted that Black women's experience of COVID-19 was shaped by the multiple oppression they experienced (Jackson and Pederson, 2020).

The authors argued that the risk of COVID-19 was amplified by the multiple other risks that Black women faced: the risks of losing their jobs or having to work as essential workers, being care givers and having direct experience of someone dying of COVID-19. A *Washington Post*-Ipsos survey found that 31 per cent of Black adults knew someone who had died of COVID-19 compared with 9 per cent of White Americans (Jackson and Pederson, 2020).

The media coverage of the impact of COVID-19 on the BAME community in the UK

In the UK, reporting of the impact of COVID-19 on the BAME community often included personal accounts of specific individuals who had suffered or died from COVID-19. In *The Guardian*, an article published on the front page of the print edition of the paper on 23 April 2020 carried the headline, 'Revealed: scale of coronavirus's deadly toll of ethnic minorities' (Barr et al, 2020a, p. 1; one online version of the article carried the headline 'Ethnic minorities dying of Covid-19 at higher rate, analysis shows', Barr et al, 2020b). The inside page story had photographs of nine ethnic minority victims alongside accounts of their lives and deaths (Barr et al, 2020a, p. 8). Another online version of the article focused on the death of 67-year-old Choudhary Aslam Wassan, a Birmingham businessman who died of COVID-19 on 29 March 2020. It was based mainly on an interview with his son, Zia Wassan. Zia felt that his father and other members of the Asian community had not been protected: 'What is happening is not normal. We 100% need answers. This is not adding up – why are so many Asian men dying. It is not normal. There is something behind this and it's my strong view that it needs to be investigated' (Parveen, 2020a).

Comment

The risk narrative that Daniel Defoe pioneered in his fictional eyewitness account of the 1665 London Plague was still evident in the media coverage of the impact of COVID-19 on vulnerable individuals. The numbers remained important; they showed heightened risk and vulnerability. But alongside the numbers were personal stories and images that helped readers identify specific victims and empathise with their suffering. Readers could make sense of the objective reality of the numbers through the emotions of friends and relatives of the victims – both their sadness at losing a loved one and their anger at the failure of those responsible to protect them.

Risk often appears as a very abstract impersonal concept, as probabilities expressed by numbers. For policy makers, it is precisely the apparent objectivity, lack of emotion and the malleability of numbers that make them so attractive. Frank, Slovic and Vastfjall (2011) observed that numbers and statistics don't bleed, and can act as 'barriers to an ethical response to suffering' (p. 609). Newcomb has argued that numbers are vulgar as they 'fail to evoke either strong affective responses that images often do or the potent feelings that go with stories' (Frank, Slovic and Vastfjall, 2011, p. 609). Narrative matrices combining quantitative data on the risks that different groups are exposed to with qualitative narratives of the ways in which COVID-19 impacted on individuals and groups provide insights into the suffering caused by the pandemic.

It is rare for policy makers to use such narratives, though the case of Captain Tom is an exception. His story can be seen in some ways as a counter-narrative, a story of heroism in face of the risks of COVID-19. It played to English nationalism and exceptionalism, referencing national unity and the 'Dunkirk spirit'.

Media stories that combined statistics with images and stories enabled viewers and readers to grasp how the pandemic was impacting on vulnerable and marginalised groups within society, such as elderly residents in care homes and front-line workers from ethnic minorities. It also provided insight into the ways in which policy makers had failed to assess the risks these groups were exposed to and provide them with adequate protection. The use of eyewitnesses creates a sense of authenticity and a sense that the reader or viewer has access to a first order direct observer, rather than relying on a second order observer and a secondhand account (Luhmann, 1993).

8

Contesting risk: conspiracy theories

Risk, broadcasting and social media

Trust, risk and communication

With the development of mass media, individuals can access a wide range of competing sources of information. Individuals have to decide which sources they trust and which they do not (Luhmann, 1993, pp 1–31). For information derived from a source that an individual has personal knowledge of, such as a friend or family, the decision whether to trust or not is shaped by the nature of the relationship. Where the information is derived from an impersonal source such as a newspaper article or a television broadcast, then decisions are shaped by more abstract criteria, such as the evaluation of the source and the extent to which a warning fits with personal experience and direct observations (Kiisel and Vihalemm, 2014).

There are problems in relying on and trusting either immediate kin and friends or the mass broadcast media. While we know the former personally and often share their values, seeing the world in similar ways, their experiences and wider knowledge are likely to be nearly as limited as ours. In contrast, while broadcasters in the mass media have access to wider sources of information, the relationship is impersonal and asymmetrical: the broadcaster has a wider range of sources but controls how they are used. The development of social media has created a new form of communication that combines features of informal communication between family and friends and more formal and structured broadcasting. For most users, social media is an online extension of their informal social networks, one in which creating and maintaining profiles establishes identity (Quinn and Papacharissi, 2014), and participation is either friendship or interest driven (Kahne and Bowyer, 2018).

The impact of social media

Individuals can use online networks to bypass or counter their normal social networks, gaining support that their friends and family disapprove of or consider risky. Fage-Butler (2017) found that pregnant women used social media networks to provide support for their decision to have a home birth when their families and professionals categorised home birth as dangerous and risky. As Jurich observes in a study of the ways in which mothers managed the risk of feeding babies with food allergies, being part of online Facebook communities enabled mothers to find solutions in real time as they received immediate responses to their posts (2021, p. 141). Although they obtained advice from doctors as well, this was a 'relatively uniform and future-oriented risk-management process' (Jurich, 2021, p. 128).

Social networks can also provide more open public communication and debate, forums within which 'networked publics' can interact (Quinn and Papacharissi, 2014). While such forums can be open, interactive and egalitarian, they can also be dominated by individuals who accumulate a substantial following, so-called influencers. When such influencers are politicians, social media take on some of the characteristic of a social movement in which a charismatic leader communicates with his or her followers. In the US, Donald Trump used social media especially Twitter, to create and connect with his supporters. His messaging was ideological and emotional, with symbols such as borders featuring prominently. This created a sense of authenticity; a sense that the reader had a direct relationship with the real Donald Trump. Shane (2018) observes that 'the typographical texture [of Trump's Tweets] tells us about Trump's personality and emotional state. It implies a speed of composition, impulsivity, and the lack of PR intervention.' Such messaging gave Trump supporters a sense of connection, belonging and purpose, important feelings that helped to counteract the isolation and loneliness that many experience in modern societies.

When social media is used by influencers, it tends to function in the same way as mass media, to broadcast messages to a wider audience. However, social media does not have the same editorial controls, checks and balances as the mass media. It does not have the traditions of journalistic practice, supervision by editors or external regulation, and it is relatively free of the pressures on the mass media – to be truthful and to appeal to wider audiences. The users of traditional media decide what content they wish to read or view, while social media use algorithms that identify users' interests and suggest items they may be interested in reading or viewing. In 2019, a Facebook researcher invented a user, Carol Smith, giving her a profile that indicated an interest in politics, parenting and Christianity, and identifying her interest in Fox News and Donald Trump. Within two days, Facebook recommended she join QAnon groups supporting conspiracy theories, and within a week her feed was full of postings from groups and pages that violated Facebook's own rules about hate speech and disinformation (Zadrozny, 2021).

Social media versus mass media

Comparisons of mass media and social media are relatively rare. One exception is de Melo and Figueiredo's (2021) analysis of reporting during the early stages of Brazilian pandemic. They evaluated news articles (18,413) and tweets (1,597,934 posted by 1,299,084 users) in the early stages of the pandemic (January–May 2020). They found that the content of the news articles and tweets covered the same five topics; the key people involved, the most important organisations, the disease categories, the symptoms and the disease. The word cloud representations of articles and tweets were similar. Both the news articles and tweets highlighted Bolsonaro and Trump, and both identified fever, cough and pain as the main symptoms of COVID-19. There was some difference in the drug category, both news articles and tweets highlighting chloroquine and hydroxychloroquine, but the newspaper articles gave prominence to vaccination (de Melo and Figueiredo, 2021, Figures 9–13). The similarity between news articles and tweets led de Melo and Figueiredo to conclude that there was cross referencing between the two types of media. They did find differences, however. The news articles tended to rely more on official sources, while tweets tended to focus on personal opinions and experiences. Tweets often took a critical position on topics, while news articles were more neutral. The issue of political polarisation was discussed in both types of media, with evidence of increasingly critical comments over time. One key issue was drug therapy, especially the Brazilian government's advocacy of chloroquine as a way of treating COVID-19.

Mistrust of the expert consensus: conspiracy theories

The media and the promotion of views critical of expert opinion

Beck (1992) and Giddens (1991) have argued that in late modern societies individuals are both more vulnerable to and more reliant on science and technology to identify and manage risks. Such reliance may create ambivalence, even a fear of science and technology. Individuals have to decide how they are going to respond to the various warnings about risk and how they are going to access the knowledge they need to manage these risks. The multiplication of experts and expertise means that in late modern society there is no longer a single authority, a single source providing explanation and guidance (Giddens, 1991, p. 195). There are 'a plurality of heterogeneous claims to knowledge, in which science does not have a privileged place' (Giddens, 1990, p. 2). There are multiple sources, often providing conflicting explanations and challenging each other. The lack of unified authority creates uncertainty and doubt, and potentially a mistrust of sources that claim authority (Giddens, 1990, p. 89).

In modern societies, individuals depend on complex technological systems, but most individuals do not have the specialist knowledge that would enable them to understand how and why such systems work (Alaszewski and Brown, 2007). The growth and fragmentation of knowledge alongside the development of error-prone complex systems has undermined the basic Enlightenment premise that knowledge will empower and liberate humanity.

Instead, as Beck has observed, 'the sources of danger are no longer ignorance but *knowledge*' (emphasis in the original, Beck, 1992, p. 183).

Burgess (2002) has noted that new technologies such as mobile phones have attracted anxiety and fear. He examined national responses to one aspect of this technology, mobile or cell phone masts. He found that in some countries there was high anxiety about and resistance to the building of such masts close to human habitations, whereas in others there were no such concerns. Burgess observed that health fears about mast emissions were triggered in the US by a 1990 lawsuit in which David Reynard claimed that his wife's cancer was caused by mobile phone radiation. Though this action and others like it failed because of lack of evidence, they attracted extensive media coverage and public interest, stimulating the growth of local groups opposing the technology. Initially, the campaigns focused on the danger to children, and in 1993 San Francisco became the first major city to ban phone masts near schools (Burgess, 2002, p. 179). Such decisions were based on the precautionary principle: there was no evidence to show mobile phone masts were dangerous but it was better to be safe than sorry.

Comment

Andrade (2020) defines conspiracy theories as 'narratives about events or situations, that allege there are secret plans to carry out sinister deeds'. Conspiracy theories can be defined as 'attempts to explain particular events or situations, as the result of the actions of a small, powerful group, with perverse intentions' (Andrade, 2020). Such theories are evident both in the Global South and the North. The identification of the malevolent 'small, powerful' group varies. In the Global South, neo-colonialism means that such groups are identified as foreign governments, aid agencies or major donors. In the Global North, conspiracy theories have become intertwined with populist politics.

Conspiracy theories in the Global South

In the Global South, rapid urbanisation combined with the slow development of infrastructure has created conditions in which infectious diseases can spread rapidly. Efforts to control outbreaks are often hampered by infodemics, defined as 'too much information including false or misleading information in digital and physical environments during a disease outbreak' (WHO, 2022). Conspiracy theories form an important part of such infodemics.

In Pakistan, conspiracy theories developed around the polio vaccination programme. As Andrade and Hussain (2018) noted, resistance to the polio vaccine is based on a theory that this programme is 'a scheme created by the United States and Israel to sterilize the Muslim population'. Andrade and Hussain (2018) traced the origin of the theory back to Nigeria in 2001, where Ibrahim Datti Ahmed, a Nigerian physician and head of the Supreme Council of Shariah of Nigeria, responded to 9/11 by publicly proclaiming that polio vaccines were 'corrupted and tainted by evildoers from America and their Western allies' and that the vaccines included anti-fertility drugs and could cause AIDS.

In Pakistan, there is a well-established resistance to vaccination programmes. It is one of the two remaining countries where polio is still endemic, mainly because of the failure of vaccination campaigns: people in Pakistan also believe in a persistent conspiracy theory that the polio vaccine is a ploy designed by the US Central Intelligence Agency to make Muslim men sterile.

In their study of COVID-19 conspiracy theories in Pakistan, Ejaz and his colleagues (2021) noted that Pakistanis have been described as receptive to conspiracy theories. An Ipsos poll in Pakistan found that a third of the respondents believed in a COVID-19 pandemic conspiracy theory (Ejaz et al, 2001, p. 165). Ejaz and his colleagues (2021, p. 165) reported that a number of such theories were circulating in 2020, including theories that:

- Bill Gates, the American philanthropist, was spreading the virus so he could profit from the sale of vaccines.
- The Israeli government was using vaccines to insert microchips into Muslims to read their thoughts.

Ittefaq, Hussain and Fatima (2020) stressed the specific cultural/religious element of some of the theories:

- COVID-19 was a plot by non-Muslims to keep believers from practising their religion and worshipping at mosques.
- COVID-19 was the product of misbehaviour by women.

Survey data from Ipsos and Gallup Pakistan in June 2020 indicated that only 3 per cent of those surveyed had no misconceptions about the virus, a third believed in conspiracy theories relating to the pandemic, and over half believed the threat was being exaggerated (Saleem, 2020).

Ejaz and his colleagues (2021) found that a major factor associated with belief in conspiracy theories was trust in social media. As Ullah (2017) has noted, politics and religion are intertwined in many Islamic countries, and social media platforms provide a means of mobilising support. For example, the power of Islamic social media was 'demonstrated in 2012 when riots broke out in the Muslim world in response to a low-budget amateurish video that insulted the Prophet Mohammed. This global upheaval ... was generated and coordinated through Islamic social media outlets' (Ullah, 2017, p. xxiv). While social media platforms are relatively recent developments

(Twitter first went online in 2006), they have grown rapidly, and in Islamic countries clerics are key influencers. In Saudi Arabia in 2017, four of the top ten Twitter accounts were clerics, with Mohammed al-Arefe who had over 17 million followers being a key influencer who was sympathetic to ISIS (Ullah, 2017, p. 10). In Pakistan, religious leaders also played a prominent role in shaping responses to the pandemic. For example, Tariq Jamal, an Islamic cleric with a strong following, claimed that 'the coronavirus is a sign of God's wrath over such sins as women dancing and dressing immodestly' (Aamir, 2020). Mufti Masood, a Islamic cleric supporting the Taliban movement in Pakistan, claimed that 'that Jews created the coronavirus for the purpose of "global governance," and that any vaccine developed will be controlled by Jews' (*Jerusalem Post* Staff, 2020).

Conspiracy theories in the Global North

Religion and conspiracy theories

The pandemic was also a fertile ground for the development of conspiracy theories in the high-income countries of the Global North. It is possible to identify a religious strand in resistance to conventional scientific explanations of the pandemic. Given the significance of Christianity in Europe and North America, one element in the conspiracy theory has been to blame rival religions, especially Islam, for the pandemic. As Awan and Khan-Williams observed in their study of posting on social media, the 'Coronavirus crisis has sparked online hate speech targeted at Muslims and an influx of Islamophobic fake news on social media sites' (Birmingham City University, 2020). When they analysed postings on Facebook, Twitter and Telegram, they found shared content indicating that Muslims were to blame for the spread of virus and that:

- Mosques were responsible for the spread of COVID-19;
- Muslims were superspreaders of the coronavirus;
- Police gave favourable treatment to Muslims out of fear of being accused of racism;
- Muslims were not observing social distancing rules. (Birmingham City University, 2020)

This religious aspect of conspiracy theories overlapped with a second element, right-wing populism. In their study of Islamophobia and the pandemic, Awan and Khan-Williams observed that 'Covid-19 has been utilised by the far-right and those who sympathise with this ideology to peddle hate, with such narratives quickly being able to penetrate the mainstream and become normalised' (Birmingham City University, 2020, p. 2). They reported that a video posted on the Telegram media site by

Tommy Robinson, a prominent UK right-wing extremist, purporting to show Muslim men leaving a mosque had been viewed over 10,000 times.

Populism and conspiracy theories

The promotion of conspiracy theories by populist leaders reflects similarities in their ideological underpinnings. Both explain misfortune and disasters as the result of the actions of small and secret malevolent groups. As Kriesi (2014) observed, the ideologies of populism draw on a basic conspiracy theory in which society is divided into 'two homogenous groups—"the people" and "the elite"', with 'the positive valorisation of "the people" combined with the denigration of "the elite"' (p. 362). The 'corrupt elite' seeking to controlling and exploit 'the pure people'. Populist leaders claim to represent the people and seek to mobilise those communities left behind or marginalised by globalisation. In the UK, for example, Boris Johnson's Brexit policies and levelling up rhetoric made inroads into 'red wall' constituencies in the north of England that traditionally supported the Labour party.

The so-called 'corrupt' elites include the political establishment, which conspiracy theorists often refer to as the hidden or 'deep state'. In the 2016 presidential election, Donald Trump's call to 'drain the swamp' was an attack on the Washington political establishment (Trump, 2016). However, 'corrupt' elites can also include technical experts and professionals. In the UK, populist Brexit campaigners attacked the unelected technocrats in the European Commission for imposing arbitrary regulations on the UK (O'Toole, 2018). When Michael Gove, a leading Brexiter, was challenged during the Brexit referendum campaign to name any economist who backed Britain's exit from the European Union, he replied that 'people in this country have had enough of experts' (Mance, 2016).

In the US, Donald Trump attacked experts and expertise at both national and international level. Nationally, he used his executive powers to limit funding to the CDC and cut the post of Director for Global Health Security and Biothreats, thereby undermining the early warning system for pandemics (Horton, 2020, p. 36). He continually criticised Anthony Fauci (uPolitics, 2020). In October 2020, Trump made the following comments:

> 'People are tired of COVID. People are saying, "Whatever, just leave us alone". People are tired of hearing Fauci and all these idiots,' said Trump. 'He's been here for, like, 500 years. He's like this wonderful sage telling us how. Fauci, if we listened to him, we'd have 700,000 [or] 800,000 deaths.' (uPolitics, 2020)

Trump was also hostile to international institutions and their experts; he was highly critical of the WHO, for example. He promoted his version of reality through his social media postings, frequently attacking conventional broadcast media with the claim that the reality they represented was 'fake news'. Trump's messages, that experts were exaggerating the threat of the virus and that public health measures were excessive, fed into the narrative that COVID-19 was either a minor illness or even a hoax.

Populist politics have stimulated a number of social movements based on conspiracy theories. Many of these predated the COVID-19 pandemic, but as the pandemic developed they absorbed it into their narratives of malevolent elites and deep states. One such movement is QAnon. The leader or leadership is anonymous, and it started as an almost completely online movement. QAnon started to attract mainstream media attention in 2018, and by 2020, following its first prediction that Hillary Clinton was about to be arrested and would flee the country, it was making multiple predictions, for example that there would be a car bomb in London around 18 February 2018 (Wikipedia, 2020). Given the movement's attacks on Hillary Clinton and other Democrats, it was endorsed by nearly 100 Republican candidates in the run-up to the 2020 election, and received presidential acknowledgement, with Donald Trump retweeting messages from QAnon followers (Kaiser, 2022).

QAnon and other right-wing conspiracy groups played an important role in resistance to public health measures that were designed to reduce the risks associated with COVID-19. When the Omicron variant was creating a new wave of infection towards the end of 2021, despite evidence that vaccination protected vulnerable people from serious illness, QAnon supporters were campaigning against vaccination. As Kaiser observed, their message was 'both clear and completely contradicted by the available evidence: they believed the pandemic was over and any mandates related to vaccines or masks were totalitarian control mechanisms that were actually killing people' (Kaiser, 2022).

The resistance was not limited to online communication, but as Mogelson (2022) has noted, the same alliance of right-wing groups that stormed Congress on 6 January 2021 to try to overturn Donald Trump's defeat was evident in earlier riots against public health measures. In Michigan in April 2020, right-wing militias reacted to the Democratic governor's extension of lockdown by initiating Operation Gridlock, a street protest that eventually spread to 30 states. On 30 April, armed protestors entered the Michigan State Capitol building, intimidating state officials and legislators.

Anxieties about science and technology

Modern medicine has developed effective technologies for preventing and managing disease. However, public understanding of how such technologies work has not kept pace with the speed of innovation. As a result, these technologies can elicit fears and anxieties that find their expression in conspiracy theories.

Such fears and anxieties are particularly evident in vaccination, the consumption or injection of material into the body to stimulate the immune system to enable it to recognise and fight specific diseases. Vaccination has been highly effective in reducing the incidence of and even eradicating diseases such as smallpox. Early forms of vaccination involved injecting live micro-organisms; for example, the smallpox vaccine is a vaccina, a poxvirus that elicits the same immune response as the smallpox virus, providing three to five years' protection (CDC, 2022a). COVID-19 vaccines are manufactured entities. The Pfizer-BioTech and Moderna vaccines use manufactured sections of mRNA (messenger ribonucleic acid) to construct different types of proteins in order to trigger the appropriate immune response inside the body (CDC, 2022b).

A vaccination involves injecting a foreign body into individuals when they are not ill. Some of those injected will experience side effects and will become ill, often mildly but occasionally seriously. The public health justification for vaccination is that it will prevent the spread of the disease, and the collective benefits outweigh the (rare) individual serious side effect. In the early 19th century, Edward Jenner popularised and gave scientific authority to vaccination as a method of preventing smallpox (Riedel, 2005). There was a lack of public understanding of how this new technology worked, resulting in mistrust and resistance to the new technology on the grounds that it involved polluting the human body by inserting impure animal material (Watson, 2019).

Smallpox vaccination is no longer contested as it has successfully eradicated the disease, but other vaccines have taken its place. In Europe and the US, 'bad science' played a role in the anti-vax movement, and social media provided a space for private discourse where such science could be communicated without being challenged and tested. In the UK, Andrew Wakefield and his scientific colleagues announced a new disease (autistic enterocolitis) that they claimed was caused by the measles, mumps and rubella (MMR) vaccine, and they published an article in *The Lancet* in February 1998. At the time, Wakefield was working with an anti-vaccine campaign group, Jabs, and was involved in a joint action by 1,500 claimants who were seeking compensation for vaccine damage to their children. Wakefield failed to disclose this conflict of interest (Editors of the Lancet, 2004). Neither Wakefield nor other researchers have been able to repeat his study, and following critical academic scrutiny, the editor of *The Lancet* withdrew the article. When Wakefield was struck off the medical register for unethical research, anti-vaxxer websites rallied to his support. The Jabs website alleged that there was an 'unrelenting barrage of anti-Wakefield propaganda in the British media' (Jabs, 2011).

The anti-vax movement maintained its hostile critique of all vaccination. On its website, Jabs published a blog that cited the danger of the flu vaccination and by implication COVID-19 vaccination (Jabs, 2020). A posting on the Jabs website was headlined: '"The Vaccines Kill Two People for Every Three Lives They Save", Says Peer-Reviewed Vaccine Study' (Jabs, 2022). Tracking the article to its sources in the journal *Vaccines* (Walach, Klement and Aukema, 2021), it is clear that the article was published on 24 June 2021, but following expressions of concern about its methodology, it was withdrawn or retracted on 2 July 2021.

After he was struck off the medical register in the UK, Wakefield moved to the US where, with his new partner, Elle Macpherson, a celebrity and supermodel, he maintained his anti-vaccination campaign. Speaking at the Health Freedom event in May 2020, he argued that: 'One of the main tenets of mandatory vaccination has been fear, and never have we seen such fear exploited in the way we do now with the coronavirus infection' (Wakefield, quoted in Carter, 2020).

This mistrust of mainstream science is grounded in a belief that it conceals the truth. This can be seen in the assertions that the manufacturers of vaccines and other 'harmful' drugs profit from the state-funded vaccination programmes. One anti-vaccination website, Learn the Risk, aimed to make the world population aware of the risks of vaccinations by 'educating people WORLDWIDE on the dangers of pharmaceutical products, including vaccines and unnecessary medical treatments — that are literally **killing** us' (emphasis in the original, Learn The Risk, n.d.).

Anti-vax sentiment is linked to a wider anxiety about the impact of modern technology. For example, the first cases of COVID-19 in China coincided with the roll-out of a new mobile phone technology, 5G, and this new technology was incorporated in conspiracy narratives. In the UK, David Icke, a former TV sports presenter, is a major promoter of conspiracy theories and 5G became part of his narrative. In a blog posted on his site, Makia Freeman asserted that in China, Wuhan was one of the first cities chosen for 5G roll-out and that the roll-out on 31 October 2019 was linked to the coronavirus outbreak beginning as 'many scientific documents on the health effects of 5G have verified that it causes flu-like symptoms' (Freeman, 2020). Freeman claimed that 5G was a military technology of a type that had caused previous disasters: 'Remember, directed energy weapons (DEW) are behind the fall of the Twin Towers on 9/11 and the fake Californian "wildfires"' (Freeman, 2020). Like many conspiracy theorists, he argued that the truth was being suppressed: 'Various independent researchers around the web, for around 2–3 weeks now, have highlighted the coronavirus-5G link despite the fact that Google (as the self-appointed NWO Censor-in-Chief) is doing its best to hide and scrub all search results showing the connection' (Freeman, 2020).

The 5G theories link to more traditional anti-technology theories, especially those around vaccination. For example, in a blog on the David Icke website, Freeman made the connection in the following way: 'If you dig deep enough, some disturbing connections arise between 5G and the men who have developed or are developing vaccines for novel viruses like ebola, zika and the new coronavirus COVID-19' (Freeman, 2020). Freeman (2020) argued that 5G is part of a conspiracy based on 'mandatory vaccine agenda, the depopulation agenda and transhumanist agenda (via DNA vaccines)'.

Factors that facilitated the spread of conspiracy theories during the pandemic

Conspiracy theories reflect a mistrust of established authority, politicians and the experts that advice the public and the development of and trust in alternative on-line communities.

Mistrust of 'official' experts

In countries with populist leaders, there was at times open conflict between politicians and health experts over the threat posed by COVID-19 and how to respond to it. Such conflict and the mixed messages associated with it created mistrust and opened up the space within which alternative narratives could flourish. This same phenomenon was observed in earlier epidemics.

In the 2014/2015 Ebola outbreak in West Africa, poor communication by governments created mistrust and a space filled by local rumours that 'the virus had been manufactured in a US military facility or that it was a plot by governments to attract foreign aid to the region' (Honigsbaum, 2020, p. 208). There was a hostile response to the foreign medical teams that were attempting to introduce public health measures, some of which undermined traditional practices and beliefs. In the early stages, these medical teams were attacked, and in one incident eight members of a delegation of government officials and medical personnel were killed (Honigsbaum, 2020, p. 207).

In the COVID-19 pandemic, poor government communication, especially the open conflict between the president and health experts in the US, created a space in which conspiracy theories could flourish (see Chapter 4).

In the UK, the House of Commons Committee on Health and Social Care and the Committee on Science and Technology highlighted the role that mistrust in government played in the development of conspiracy theories, noting that: 'Lower levels of public trust and understanding of the regulations also created a gap into which misinformation was able to spread' (2021, para 148). They drew attention to ways in which 'the inconsistency in Government messaging after the first wave of the pandemic was also damaging to public trust in official information' (2021, para 147). They noted the ways in which public perceptions that key government figures had broken lockdown rules contributed to the undermining of public trust (2021, para 147).

In their qualitative study of trust and mistrust in experts in four relatively new European democracies (Czech Republic, Hungary, Poland, and Serbia) during the early stages of the pandemic, Mihelj, Kondor and Štětka (2022) found that trust in experts was a major concern for the participants in their study. Most were willing to trust experts because they were experts; that is, they were knowledgeable. For example, 'Two Serbian participants explained that they trust experts because they know more about the virus … while a Czech participant explained his trust with reference to general trust in science and scientific facts' (Mihelj, Kondor and Štětka, 2022, p, 303). This general trust did not extend to all experts. In all four countries, the governments included right-wing populist politicians. As Mihelji and his colleagues observed, in some former communist countries there was mistrust of populist governments and a concern that they had politicised the pandemic and used it as a way of extending their power and restricting civil liberties. This mistrust of politicians spread to experts who were closely associated with the governments, especially in Serbia and Hungary, where there was mistrust of experts on government-appointed national crisis teams.

Participants' trust was also undermined if and when there was disagreement among experts. In the Czech Republic, there was a debate between medical experts advocating lockdown measures and those advocating a herd immunity strategy. One Czech reflected on this debate in the following way: 'And now we have here this pandemic and half of the epidemiologists say let's keep lockdown and the other [half] is for letting the virus go into the population. So, what is a common man to think? Maybe it is better to pray' (Mihelj, Kondor, and Štětka, 2022, p, 306).

Participants' trust was also influenced by sources of expert opinion, especially the type of media outlet experts used. Most participants in the study encountered experts through official government sources, especially broadcast briefings that involved medical experts (Mihelj, Kondor, and Štětka, 2022, p, 307). Their response to such broadcasts was influenced by their political views and their perception of the integrity of the experts. In Hungary and Serbia, where there was mistrust of experts in the national crisis team and their contribution to mainstream, pro-government news media, participants tended to use alternative sources to access expert opinions, especially social media (Mihelj, Kondor, and Štětka, 2022, p, 308). In Poland, the mass media was polarised between pro- and anti-government outlets, with readers and viewers divided along similar lines. Some of the Polish participants in the study judged the independence and trustworthiness of experts according to 'whether they appeared in media aligned with their political convictions' (Mihelj, Kondor, and Štětka, 2022, p, 307).

Trust in and reliance on the social media as a source of expertise

As Mihelj, Kondor, and Štětka (2022) observed, individuals who mistrust experts, especially those whose integrity was seen as compromised by their links to national politics, look for alternative sources of expertise. This could be local experts they personally know and trust, but more often they access alternative expert opinion through social media. Thus, several participants who were university educated and mistrusted government sources used social media to find trustworthy foreign experts (2022. p. 308). Mihelj, Kondor, and Štětka noted that participants in their study found social media more accessible and were particularly attracted to YouTube, which combined audio-visual communication with an absence of editorial, providing directness and creating a sense of authenticity (2022, p. 310).

In their study of ways in which Twitter in particular shaped narratives in France on COVID-19 vaccines, Faccin et al (2022) observed that 'The mobilization of vaccine-critical activists is another factor that meshes with the previous ones, as these activists draw on distrust in public deciders and on discourses downplaying the epidemic to convince the largest possible public not to take this particular vaccine and join their cause' (2022, p. 2).

On Twitter, discussions are initiated by an initial posting that stimulates responses, thereby creating an avalanche of retweeting so that information is spread through a network of contacts. Faccin and colleagues noted that the volume of tweets and retweets fluctuated in response to a trigger event or announcement. They identified ten such triggers between February 2020 and May 2021, including 'COVID-19 came from a lab experiment' (2 February 2020), report of adverse events and a death in COVID-19 clinical trials (6 June 2020), first appearance of #stopdictaturesanitaire (11 October 2020) and the suspension by Danish authorities of the AstraZeneca COVID-19 vaccine (10 March 2021) (Faccin et al, 2022).

They explored the pattern in which tweets spread, identifying online communities or retweet networks in which there were established links between users who retweeted to each other. Such communities could form self-contained bubbles when there was little or no retweeting outside the established boundary of the community or they could be more open. Faccin et al (2022) identified 30 larger communities who posted and shared tweets about COVID-19 and COVID-19 vaccines. Most of these communities represented established communication groups, including government representatives, public institutions, medical doctors, French and international news media and media aggregators or French web influencers. There were also far right groups, far left groups and trade unions (see Figure 4, Faccin et al, 2022. p. 11).

There were differences in the ways in which these groups signposted their tweets using hashtags. The most prominent hashtags used by established communication groups were those relating to government and public health. They also used the hashtag #antivax, not as a way of marking self-identity but more as a form of media commentary. In contrast, right-wing communities used hashtags highlighting their hostility towards public health measures, for example, #nopasssanitaire and #dictaturesanitaire; their criticism of vaccination, for example, #bigpharma; and their interest in alternative treatments such as #hydroxychloroquine. They tended to avoid institutional hashtags such as #macron or #gouvernment and public health hashtags, for example, #vaccinecovid and #vaccinezvous. They also referenced the French populist protest movement, the Gilets Jaunes.

The left-wing community also retweeted hashtags critical of COVID-19, emphasising the critical role of pharmaceutical companies with the hashtag #bigpharma. However, unlike the right-wing communities, they also used hashtags relating to contemporary politics and social movements. This reflected the different ways in which the two communities operated. The right-wing communities formed closed bubbles. While these bubbles absorbed vaccine-critical tweets from other communities, they tended to act as echo chambers, with retweets within the community. In the left-wing communities there was more regular retweeting outside the community, so while the left wing communities absorbed less anti-vax content, they were actually more active in distributing it and had 'a higher capacity to spread this kind of information to a larger public' (Faccin et al, 2022. p. 12).

Right wing communities only broke out of their echo chambers when there was a COVID-related controversy that attracted wider political and media attention. Faccin et al (2022, p. 15) reflected on the ways in which the hydroxychloroquine controversy in March 2020 enabled right-wing communities in France to reach a wider community. The debate engaged the mainstream media for several weeks, and centred on whether the public could trust experts and the government about clinical research, the severity of COVID-19 and the probity of researchers, public agencies and the government. As Faccin et al observed this controversy, and the ways in which right-wing communities exploited it to reach a wider audience 'should remind us that doubts regarding vaccines and criticism of vaccines are never just about vaccines. They are also about trust in public health authorities, in agencies in charge of authorizing medical products and monitoring their safety, in mainstream scientific research and even about politics' (2022, p. 15).

Comment

In late modern society, there is reasonable scepticism about some of the claims made by science and technology. For example, pharmaceutical companies that have their research and development facilities in high-income countries advertise and promote their products, making substantial profits, and on occasion their products have substantial negative externalities in ways that are shocking and create widespread suffering. Thalidomide was used to treat nausea in pregnant women and resulted in serious birth defects (Kim and Scialli, 2011). Conspiracy theorists take some of these reasonable doubts, extend them and weave them into theories that deny the benevolent motives of governments and experts or express the view that conventional therapies such as vaccination are harmful. In seeking to refute conspiracy theories, government agencies seldom address the wider and more reasonable doubts about science and technology.

The internet provides the medium in which conspiracy theories can develop relatively uncontested. Lockdown provided a stimulus. Individuals were cut off from their normal social networks and sources of reality, and as many experienced increased anxiety and uncertainty, pursuing conspiracies could be a satisfying pastime. Conspiracy theorists adopted the rhetoric of science, claiming to use research to search for the truth – but given the ways in which social media creates communities of like-minded individuals who reinforce each other's beliefs, these claims were not subject to rigorous scrutiny (Wong, 2020).

Case Study 10: Resistance to wearing masks in the US

Transmission of the COVID-19 and risk minimisation

One way of minimising the risk of COVID-19 is to interrupt the transmission of the virus. As I note in Chapter 6, at the start of the pandemic there was a scientific consensus that SARS-CoV-2 was transmitted by droplet infection. The consensus among public health experts (apart from those in Japan) was that the best way for individuals to protect themselves was to focus on personal hygiene such as hand washing and cleaning surfaces and to avoid close personal contact. In the early stages of the pandemic, the WHO recommended that only individuals who were ill or were caring for individuals with COVID-19 should wear face masks. The WHO argued that there was not enough evidence to indicate that healthy people should wear masks to reduce transmission of the virus (BBC, 2020d). However on 5 June, the WHO director-general updated WHO guidance, recommending that:

> In areas with widespread transmission, WHO advises medical masks for all people working in clinical areas of a health facility, not only workers dealing with patients with COVID-19. … in areas with community transmission, we advise that people aged 60 years or over, or those with underlying conditions, should wear a medical mask in situations where physical distancing is not possible. … In light of evolving evidence, WHO advises that governments should encourage the general public to wear masks where there is widespread transmission and physical

distancing is difficult, such as on public transport, in shops or in other confined or crowded environments. (Ghebreyesus, 2020b)

In the UK, the advice changed with the understanding of how the virus was transmitted. In his statement on 12 March 2020, as the first cases were announced, Prime Minister Boris Johnson warned the population about the virus and stated that 'it is still vital, perhaps more vital than ever – that we remember to wash our hands (Gov.UK, 2020a). On 16 March, he again highlighted the dangers of COVID-19 and introduced measures to increase overall social distancing, advocating minimal social contact for individuals in high-risk categories and noting that 'It is far more now than just washing your hands – though clearly washing your hands remains important' (Gov.UK, 2020b). In autumn 2020, as the second wave developed, the government added mask wearing to the list of recommended protections. Chris Whitty, the CMO, summarised the advice in the following way: ' "Hands. Face. Space" emphasises important elements of the guidance we want everybody to remember: wash your hands regularly, use a face covering when social distancing is not possible and try to keep your distance from those not in your household' (Gov.UK, 2020c).

In the US, the CDC was also advocating mask wearing as a way of interrupting transmission by November 2020. The CDC posted guidance on its website under the slogan '**WEAR A MASK**, PROTECT OTHERS', with photos of six individuals from diverse backgrounds wearing masks (emphasis in the original, CDC, 2020b). The CDC recommended that: 'people wear masks in public settings, like on public and mass transportation, at events and gatherings, and anywhere they will be around other people' (CDC, 2020b). By April 2021, the CDC had updated its guidance, recommending that everyone aged two years or older should wear a mask when in public, especially when on public transport, and should wear one in private homes if there was a person present who was not a member of that household or had tested positive for COVID-19 (CDC, 2021f).

Resistance to mask wearing

In the US and Europe, in contrast to Japan, there was no tradition of mask wearing in public spaces, and recommendations to wear masks in such spaces met with resistance. Part of this resistance was linked to conspiracy theories. Some media celebrities used their substantial online fan base to promote resistance to mask wearing. For example, Ian Brown, the frontman of the UK pop group, the Stone Roses, posted a series of (now deleted) tweets in which he likened coronavirus to the common cold, suggested the crisis was 'planned and designed to make us digital slaves', and linked the virus to a fraud. One of his tweets in September 2020 read: 'NO LOCKDOWN

NO TESTS NO TRACKS NO MASKS NO VAX #researchanddestroy' (Daly, 2020).

In the US, mask wearing became entangled in the presidential election campaign, with Donald Trump refusing to wear a mask and ridiculing mask wearers, including Joe Biden, the Democratic candidate. Donald Trump displayed his rejection of masks with typical theatricality. When he returned from hospital on 6 October 2020 after his treatment for COVID-19, he arrived wearing a mask, which he removed with a flourish for the TV cameras (YouTube, 2020d).

At the start of the pandemic, Anthony Fauci did not recommend masks for the general public, but as the supply increased and the pandemic spread so his advice changed. In a virtual panel conference with public health experts in Australia, Fauci commended Australia and New Zealand for tackling the pandemic well, and commented: 'I would like to say the same for the United States, but the numbers speak for themselves' (Thorne, 2020). Fauci identified the lack of mask wearing as a major cause of the spread of infection in the US. He observed that if you watched TV images of life in the US 'you'd see people crowded at bars with no masks, just essentially causing superspreading' (Thorne, 2020). Fauci noted the mask wearing in the US had shifted from being a public health issue to being a political issue, and he found the vitriol aimed at mask-wearers extraordinary. He found it a painful experience 'as a physician, a scientist and a public health person – to see such divisiveness centred around a public health issue' (Thorne, 2020).

Risk implications

With the growth of scientific knowledge, experts have developed sophisticated technologies that have enabled them to rapidly understand and provide ways of managing existing and new dangers such as infectious diseases. Following the Spanish flu pandemic, it took over 80 years to identify the genetic structure of the virus; in 2020, it took scientists weeks to acquire the same knowledge about SARS-CoV-2. Paradoxically, such progress has not increased public trust in scientific knowledge. Alongside the growth of scientific knowledge has been the growth of alternative conspiracy theories that identify science as the main risk, and which advocate resistance to preventative measures such as vaccination and mask wearing.

Comment

The growth of conspiracy theories has been a marked phenomenon in the 21st century, facilitated by the development of online communities of conspiracy theorists. Social media platforms have recognised the dangers this presents to public discourses and taken actions to limit their growth (Wong,

2020). However, the pandemic has provided a stimulus to the development of such theories thanks to increased spare time, reduced normal social interaction and support from populist politicians such as Donald Trump.

As I observe in Chapter 4, political leaders adopted very different communication strategies. Those such as Jacinda Ahearn (New Zealand), Scott Morrison (Australia) and Giuseppe Conte (Italy) were quick to endorse conventional medical assessments of the risks posed by SARS-CoV-2 and the most effective way of mitigating the risks. In contrast, other especially populist leaders contested expert risk assessment and public health advice. For example, in the US, President Trump deliberately stoked controversy and gave 'dog whistle' support to various COVID-19 conspiracy theories. While the UK's Boris Johnson claimed to be following expert advice, he was slow to react. There was a public perception that he did not listen to experts in how to handle the virus and that, like Trump, he had a reputation for not being open and honest (Jennings et al, 2020, p. 25). The differences in approach impacted in trust in institutions. In a study of public opinion in Australia, Italy, the UK and USA during the pandemic, Jennings and his colleagues found the lowest level of trust in government in the USA (34 per cent) with the highest in Australia (52 per cent) and the UK (42 per cent) and Italy (39 per cent) falling in between. Similarly, trust in the country's health-care system was lowest in the USA (47 per cent), and higher in the UK (82 per cent), Italy (73 per cent) and Australia (72 per cent). It was also reflected in public assessment of the performance of leaders, with more than half of the respondents in the survey seeing Scott Morrison (66 per cent) and Giuseppe Conte (50 per cent) handling the COVID-19 pandemic competently and less than half seeing Johnson (37 per cent) and Trump (35 per cent) doing so (see Table 5 in Jennings et al, 2020, p. 24). Trust in institutions and leaders shaped individuals' willingness to accept the reality and seriousness of the COVID-19 pandemic. In the UK, Italy and Australia, approximately a quarter of respondents perceived that the media exaggerated the extent of the COVID-19 outbreak, whereas in the USA it was nearly 40 per cent (see Figure 12 in Jennings et al, 2020, p. 21). As Jenkins and his colleagues observed, 'Americans appear to be in the midst of a crisis of faith in their government – reflecting the country's failure to get to grips with the coronavirus and President Trump's divisive leadership throughout the crisis' (2020, p. 21). This provided an environment suited to the development of a variety of conspiracy theories.

9

Hindsight: inquiries and the blame game

Risk as a way of allocating blame for misfortune

Analysing risk is generally seen as a way of predicting and managing the future, but it can also be used to explain what went wrong in the past (Bernstein, 1996, p. 48; Douglas 1990, p. 5) and as a way of identifying failings and allocating blame. As Douglas (1992) observed, 'under the banner of risk reduction, a new blaming system has replaced the former system based on religion and sin' (p. 16). In the case of collective disasters, there is pressure to identify why risks were not foreseen and mitigated.

Inquiries, risk and blame

With the development of improved science and technology, governments can reassure their citizens that '[m]ost accidents are preventable' (Department of Health, 1993, p. 9). If this is the case, then disasters such as COVID-19 'are the outcome of poorly managed risks, rather than the inevitable misfortunes that we must all suffer from time to time' (Green, 1999, p. 25). Given that COVID-19 has affected different countries in different ways and the ways it spread and affected human populations was shaped by human decisions, it can be seen as a man-made disaster, especially in those countries with high infection and death rates.

One mechanism for examining why those involved failed to identify the risks is through a public inquiry. Such inquiries involve:

- Admission of the failure of normal decision making: Some events are considered so shocking and such an existential threat, such as the terrorist attacks in the US on 11 September 2001, that there is immediate and unanimous agreement that they need to be investigated. The 9/11 attacks were followed almost immediately by a bipartisan inquiry of the Intelligence Committees of the Senate and House of Representatives, which published its report on 10 December 2002 (Joint Inquiry, 2002). However, governments are often reluctant to admit they have failed to protect citizens, so it may require considerable pressure to persuade them to appoint an inquiry. In the UK, when a dredger, the *Bowbelle*, hit and sunk a pleasure boat, the *Marchioness*, on 20 August 1989, killing 51 of the 130 on board the *Marchioness*, the survivors and relatives of the deceased were unhappy with the initially limited investigations. After ten years of campaigning, the Secretary of State agreed to establish a full public inquiry (Clarke et al, 2001).

- Creating an arm's-length mechanism: To gain credibility and legitimacy, inquiries need to be seen as independent from the government, especially when the failures they are asked to investigate may have been caused by government actions or inactions. To ensure that inquiries are credible, they are usually chaired by independent authoritative figures, such as senior retired judges, are given broad terms of reference and the powers of a court, which allow them, for example, to summon and question witnesses and access documents. Such public inquiries are expensive and time consuming.

- Use of hindsight to identify how and why there was a failure to identify risk: Inquiries use the knowledge gained from hindsight to identify missed opportunities. The Joint Inquiry into 9/11 identified the ways in which warning signals were repeatedly ignored (Joint Inquiry, 2002, Finding 5). Similarly, the Canadian Commission established to investigate the SARS outbreak in Ontario noted that the Commission could and did use hindsight, but 'those who fought SARS did not have [the benefit of hindsight] as they faced a new and unknown disease' (Campbell, 2006a, p. 19).

- Closure for survivors: Increasingly, inquiry reports recognise and seek to address the suffering and distress of victims and their families by providing detailed evidence of the circumstances to facilitate catharsis. The inquiry team investigating the sinking of the *Marchioness* stated that: 'No-one who has attended this inquiry could fail to have been affected by the emotion and strong feelings which the events of 20th August 1989 and its aftermath have engendered. We certainly have … we can only hope that this inquiry will have played some small part in helping [the survivors] to put this appalling tragedy behind them' (Clarke et al, 2001, para. 40.73).

- Learning exercise to avoid a repetition: In Canada, the SARS Commission focused on the lessons that could be learnt from the failure to contain the outbreak, and how similar failures could be prevented in the future (Campbell, 2006b, p. 1155).

- Allocation of responsibility and blame: While inquiries focus on finding out what happened and preventing it happening again, they often identify individual and organisational failure to ascertain risks and allocate blame for such failure. For example, in the UK, the inquiry into paediatric surgery at Bristol Royal Infirmary argued that information about risky practice at Bristol Royal Infirmary was available from 1984 but those individuals who could and should have taken action chose not to. The Inquiry blamed and made adverse comments about five professionals in the Infirmary and three outside (BRI Inquiry, 2001, p. 10).

Anticipating inquiries, deflecting blame

It was clear from an early stage of the COVID-19 pandemic that 'when the time was right', in most democratic countries, there would be some sort of public or independent inquiry. These would examine how and in what ways the actions of governments and other agencies contributed to the excess death rate, what mistakes were made, who was responsible for them and how such mistakes could be avoided in the future. In October 2020, the retired head of the UK civil service, Lord Sedwill, acknowledged that an inquiry was inevitable and that 'whenever it comes will need to address two big questions, one is whether our decisions were taken at the right time, and the second big question is … what capabilities the state had …' (BBC, 2020e).

Some policy makers have tried to protect themselves from future blame. Donald Trump sought to deflect the blame for the pandemic onto experts and outsiders. In his White House press briefing on 14 April 2020, he attacked and blamed international experts (the WHO) and the Chinese for allowing COVID-19 to become a pandemic, saying:

> Today I'm instructing my administration to halt funding of the World Health Organization while a review is conducted to assess the World Health Organization's role in severely mismanaging and covering up the spread of the coronavirus. Everybody knows what's going on there. … Had the WHO done its job to get medical experts into China to objectively assess the situation on the ground and to call out China's lack of transparency, the outbreak could have been contained at its source, with very little death… (Trump, 2020)

The initial inquiries into the response of policy makers to the pandemic

Policy makers' reluctance to have their decisions scrutinised by public inquiries has not prevented the establishment of a series of regional, national and international inquiries into the handling of the pandemic.

As Griglio (2020) has noted, the pandemic has changed the ways in which many governments operate, and in particular has changed the relationship between executive and legislative branches of government. During the pandemic, executives tended to marginalise legislatures. Their normal operations were difficult to sustain during peak waves of the pandemic as social distancing rules prevented the necessary face-to-face interactions. One way of adapting to this disruption was to use legislative committees to maintain oversight of executive actions through targeted inquiries. While these committees did not have the judicial power of public inquires to summon and question witnesses or to access key documents, they could act quickly and informally, producing rapid critical comment (Griglio, 2020, p. 62).

France

On 25 March 2020, the National Assembly through its Law Committee established a fact-finding mission involving all political parties and committee in the Assembly to monitor government pandemic policies. The mission's first public meeting on 1 April 2020 was a hearing with the Minister of Health and the prime minister. The mission worked through video conferencing with direct streaming to the public (Griglio, 2020, p. 61). Initially the President of the Assembly, a member of the president's party, chaired the mission, so scrutiny of government policy was limited. However, the lower house, the Senate, in which the government did not have a majority, set up its own inquiry on 30 June 2020 into the government's preparedness, the management of the crisis and France's response compared with other countries (Derosier and Toulemonde, 2020, pp. 9–10).

Brazil

In April 2021, the Congress initiated an inquiry into the ways in which the president, Jair Bolsonaro, and his government managed the COVID-19 pandemic. The Inquiry was undertaken by 11 senators and focused on why the death rate had been so high in Brazil. It examined the management of the pandemic in particular detail: why the president sacked three health ministers before appointing Eduardo Pazuello, an army general with no public health experience; why the government failed to impose lockdowns or promote social distancing; why the health-care systems in the Amazon collapsed in January 2021; and why the government failed to source enough COVID-19 vaccines to protect the population (Phillips, 2021)? The inquiry published its report in October 2021 based on a 7–4 majority. It blamed Bolsonaro, stating that he was 'the main person responsible for the errors committed by the federal government during the pandemic' (Álvares and Jeanet, 2021). It agreed to call for Bolsonaro's prosecution on a range of charges, including misuse of public funds and crimes against humanity. Given that the Prosecutor-General was a Bolsonaro appointment, such a prosecutions was highly unlikely. However, this was anticipated by the authors of the report, who were interested in preventing Bolsonaro's re-election in the 2022 presidential elections.

UK

In the UK, policy makers acknowledged at the start of the pandemic that it would be important to have a public inquiry to learn lessons. In a press briefing on 30 April 2020, Chris Whitty, the CMO, noted that while it was important to learn lessons, this should be done at some point in the future when the pandemic was over, stating that 'you must learn lessons at the right point but what you don't do frankly is do that in the middle of something' (YouTube, 2020b). Despite pressure from the opposition political parties, groups representing bereaved families and professional associations, the prime minister did not announce the appointment of an independent public inquiry until 12 May 2021. He delayed appointing the chair, a retired judge, Baroness Heather Hallett, until 15 December 2021. She indicated that she would consult with the families of the bereaved before finalising the terms of reference for the inquiry, and that it was unlikely that work would begin until the summer of 2022 (Gov.UK, 2021h).

The delay in appointing the UK's public inquiry did not prevent parliamentary committees from undertaking their own inquiries. In its published list of pandemic inquiries, the UK Parliament lists 57 inquiries and 63 reports (UK Parliament, 2021). These tended to focus on the specific policy remits of each committee. An exception to this was the Health Committee and Science and Technology Committee joint inquiry into the overall government response to the pandemic. The committees questioned key participants in 11 oral sessions mainly in October to December 2020 and received written evidence from individuals and organisations (House of Commons, Health and Social Care Committee and Science and Technology Committee, 2021b, S1 paras 1–3). Some sessions attracted media attention. For example, the prime minister's former chief adviser Dominic Cummings gave the committees graphic insight into the confused initial response to the virus:

> When the public needed us most, the Government failed. I would like to say to all the families of those who died unnecessarily how sorry I am for the mistakes that were made, and for my own mistakes at that.
>
> Regarding the beginning of this crisis, yes, you are right that I, like many people, had talked about this before. When it started in January, I did think in part of my mind, 'Oh my goodness – is this it? Is this what people have been warning about all this time?' However, at the time PHE [Public Health England] here and the WHO and the CDC – generally speaking, organisations across the western world – were not ringing great alarm bells about it. I think in retrospect it is completely obvious that many, many institutions failed on this early question.
>
> I can't remember the precise date, but the truth is that I think the Taiwanese Government basically hit the panic button on something like new year's eve of 2019. That might not be the exact date, but within a few days. They put into effect a plan that they had figured

out from having been terrified of previous outbreaks, like SARS and whatnot. They immediately closed the borders, they produced various new quarantine systems, they did a whole bunch of things right off the bat in January, but I think it is obvious that the western world, including Britain, just completely failed to see the smoke and to hear the alarm bells in January. (House of Commons, Health and Social Care Committee and Science and Technology Committee, 2021a, Q944)

Even though the committees were made up of politicians from the ruling and opposition parties, they were able to publish an agreed report on 12 October 2021. One strategy for achieving this consensus was to highlight the importance of learning lessons rather than allocating blame. Another strategy was to allocate credit where the committee felt it was due. The committees praised:

- The government, for its foresight in investing in vaccine research and production, and Sir Patrick Vallance for initiating the Vaccine Task Force, which brought together key participants under 'the bold, authoritative leadership of Kate Bingham' (House of Commons, Health and Social Care Committee and Science and Technology Committee, 2021b, Executive Summary, para 20). Over 80 per cent of the adult population in the UK was vaccinated by September 2021.
- Health care providers, for the rapid reprovisioning of the NHS with expansion of ventilator and ICU capacity.
- Health researchers, for their research on vaccines and on evaluating treatment, showing the effectiveness of dexamethasone and the ineffectiveness of hydrochloroquine.
- The UK regulatory bodies, the MRHA and JCVI, who 'approached their crucial remit with authority and creativity' (House of Commons, Health and Social Care Committee and Science and Technology Committee, 2021b, Executive Summary, para 19), enabling the UK to become the first country to approve a COVID-19 vaccine.
- The Secretary of State for Health and Social Care, Matt Hancock, who had been criticised for setting an over-ambitious target of 100,000 COVID-19 tests a day. The committees observed that this target stimulated a rapid expansion of testing capacity, but observed that it was a failure of collective decision making that the policy relied on Hancock's personal initiative.

The committees were highly critical of the government's response to and management of the pandemic, especially at the start:

- The government failed to frame the new virus correctly. The committees noted that 'The UK's pandemic planning was too narrowly and inflexibly based on a flu model, which failed to learn the lessons from SARS, MERS and Ebola. The result was that whilst our pandemic planning had been globally acclaimed, it performed less well than other countries when it was needed most' (House of Commons, Health and Social Care Committee and Science and Technology Committee, 2021b, Executive Summary, para 1).

- The government failed to prevent the spread of the virus. A fatalistic approach was adopted, accepting that it was impossible to prevent the spread of the virus. The government did not consider or learn from the 'more emphatic and rigorous approach to stopping the spread of the virus as adopted by many East and South East Asian countries', and effectively accepted a herd immunity strategy (House of Commons, Health and Social Care Committee and Science and Technology Committee, 2021b, Executive Summary, para 2).

- The government failed to critically question scientific advice during the first three months of the pandemic. Despite predictions of high death rates, policy makers did not challenge the advice that there was no effective way of controlling the spread of the virus until it was too late and the NHS was being overwhelmed. The scientific guidance lacked transparency and failed to consider approaches that were being taken elsewhere.

- The government failed to understand that lockdown was inevitable, delaying it as long as possible. In the absence of other effective measures (border controls, effective case isolation and a developed test and trace system), lockdown was the only way of limiting the harm caused by COVID-19. When the UK government finally adopted lockdown in March 2020, 'it was because of domestic concern about the NHS being overwhelmed rather than a serious decision to follow emerging international best practice' (House of Commons, Health and Social Care Committee and Science and Technology Committee, 2021b, Executive Summary, para 6).

- The government failed to develop systems to effectively monitor the virus. The committees noted that community testing was abandoned at an early stage of the pandemic; that 'A country with a world-class expertise in data analysis should not have faced the biggest health crisis in a hundred years with virtually no data to analyse'; and that government agencies failed to share what data there was (House of Commons, Health and Social Care Committee and Science and Technology Committee, 2021b, Executive Summary, para 3).

- The government failed to develop an effective trace and test system, with the existing system being abandoned at the start of the pandemic. Although scientists in the UK developed a test for COVID-19 in January 2020, this did not lead to an effective test and trace system being set up during the first year of the pandemic. By the time such a system was established, new infections were running at 2,000 a day. The system failed to control the spread of the virus and failed to prevent further lockdowns. It was initially highly centralised, bypassing established local public health facilities, and it took over a year to develop an effective system that was led locally but had central capacity to deal with surges in infection.

- The government failed to protect the population of the UK. In the first year of the pandemic, 'the UK did significantly worse in terms of COVID-19 deaths than many countries – especially compared to those in East Asia even though they were much closer geographically to where the virus first appeared' (House of Commons, Health and Social Care Committee and Science and Technology Committee, 2021b, Executive Summary).
- The government failed to protect vulnerable residents of care homes. When the government needed to free up capacity in the NHS to prevent hospitals being overwhelmed, the rapid discharge from hospitals into care homes without proper testing or rigorous isolation caused preventable deaths.
- The government failed to protect people from BAME communities, who were at risk because of increased exposure to COVID-19. When working in front-line roles, they often experienced difficulties in accessing PPE.
- The government failed to protect people with learning disabilities and autistic people, whose relatives were unable to visit and advocate for them if they were admitted to hospital, and were inappropriately given do not resuscitate notices.

Comment

While the virus was still spreading round the globe, the actions and inactions of governments were already coming under scrutiny. Inquiries were set up, especially in legislatures in democratic countries that had a duty to oversee the executive. Political leaders were aware of such scrutiny, and responded by seeking to present their actions in the best possible light or by trying to deflect blame.

Case Study 11: The Ischgl and Paznaun valley inquiry

In this case study, I focus on one of the first independent inquiries, a small-scale regional inquiry that reported quickly. It was set up on 14 May 2020 and reported on 12 October 2020 (Hersche et al, 2020). The inquiry focused on the events that took place over a short period of time in a ski resort (Ischgl) in the Paznaun valley in Austria.

Pressure for an inquiry

By the summer of 2020, it had become clear that the European Alpine ski resorts had played a key role in the transmission of the virus from China into

Europe. Media coverage of the events in Ischgl suggested that the authorities had sought to protect the local tourist industry by covering up evidence that the virus was in the valley, allowing infected tourists to leave and spread the infection. The resort has been linked to infections in 45 countries, and a consumer rights group had decided to take legal action against the Austrian authorities (BBC, 2020f). The regional governor of the Tyrol responded to these criticisms by appointing a panel to investigate and report on what happened in the valley.

The setting up and operation of the inquiry

On 14 April 2020, the regional government set up a commission of independent experts chaired by Dr Ronald Rohrer, a former supreme court judge, 'to provide a comprehensive, transparent and independent evaluation of the management of the COVID-19 pandemic in Tyrol' (Rohrer, 2020, p. 1). The commission was a committee of experts who conducted a behind-closed-doors investigation. It was to examine and report on all the measures taken by local agencies in the Tyrol, but its terms of reference did not include an examination of the role of national politicians and authorities. The commission interviewed 53 representatives of various authorities and agencies in Tyrol and accessed 5,789 pages of documents. It reported to the Tyrolean Parliament in October 2020 (Hersche et al, 2020; Rohrer, 2020).

Findings

The commission began by identifying the key events and dates (Hersche et al, 2020, pp. 13–14, see Table 9.1).

What went wrong and whose fault was it?

The commission exonerated local agencies from the main accusation that they had acted under pressure from the local tourist industry. It found that the agencies' decisions were 'made on their own initiative and without pressure from a third party' (Rohrer, 2020, p. 3). It was observed that the agencies were making decisions in challenging circumstances (Rohrer, 2020, p. 3). Despite being explicitly prohibited from allocating blame, the commission did so, finding that local agencies hesitated and failed to act promptly and effectively. As soon as there was evidence of community transmission, they should have issued warnings and taken measures to restrict social interactions. Instead, they decided to wait and see while issuing reassuring messages. The commission noted that the local agencies were working within the framework of existing administrative laws. These were outdated, and the Federal Ministry responsible for health had failed to 'publish the revised

Table 9.1: Timeline for COVID-19-related events in Paznaun valley and Ischgl (February and March 2020)

Date	Event
26 February	Icelandic tourist in Ischgl developed symptoms of COVID-19.
29 February	11 Icelandic tourists flew home and some developed symptoms.
4 March	Icelandic authorities reported eight cases on the international Early Warning and Response System.
5 March	Icelandic authorities reported a further six cases, and three Norwegian students who had visited the après-ski bar in Ischgl tested positive. Local agencies started tracking and tracing contacts, but issued a reassuring statement that community transmission was unlikely.
7 March	Waiter from the après-ski bar tested positive.
8 March	Local agencies issued another statement that community transmission was unlikely.
9 March	Fourteen employees and one guest of the après-ski bar tested positive.
13 March	The state governor announced that the skiing season would end on 15 March. The Austrian chancellor announced the imposition of quarantine in the Paznaun valley and neighbouring resorts. A panicked and disorderly evacuation of the Paznaun valley ensued.

pandemic plan despite early knowledge of the risk of infection' (Rohrer, 2020, p. 4). The commission concluded that 'the district administrative authorities were not supported in their decision making and that the necessary rapid intervention was hindered' (Rohrer, 2020, p. 4). National authorities also shared responsibility with the local agencies for the failure to end the skiing season and evacuate all tourists and non-local workers in a timely, orderly and safe manner. They failed to communicate with local agencies, and the federal chancellor's public statement contributed to the disorderly evacuation of the valley (Rohrer, 2020, p. 3).

Risk implications

When setting up the commission, the Tyrolean authorities sought to limit its scope. By stipulating that it should be made up of technical experts, lay representatives were excluded, and the scope of the inquiry was effectively limited to the technical aspects of risk, excluding its emotional and moral dimensions. The authorities also sought to avoid the allocation of blame. This was only partially successful. Although the commission concentrated on technical issues, it also allocated blame to both local agencies and the national government. Using hindsight, the commission identified the ways in which Austrian authorities had failed to effectively identify, respond to and communicate risk, thereby allowing the virus to spread to other countries.

Case Study 12: The WHO inquiries

On 19 May 2020, the 73rd Meeting of the World Health Assembly, the constituent body of the WHO, initiated two inquiries into COVID-19. The assembly asked the Director-General to set up an inquiry into 'the zoonotic source of the virus and the route of introduction to the human population' (WHA, 2020, para 9(6)) and also to set up a broader inquiry into the international response to the pandemic and the role of the WHO in coordinating that response (WHA, 2020, para 9(10)).

Pressure for the inquiries

As an agency of the United Nations, WHO has a responsibility for identifying threats to global health and warning constituent states of new and emerging dangers. By May 2020, it was clear that warnings issued by the WHO had failed to halt the spread of COVID-19, and apart from in a few countries in and around the western Pacific rim, most countries were experiencing widespread community transmission and rising death rates as health-care systems were overwhelmed.

In the blame game that developed, the WHO was criticised, particularly by Donald Trump. He was campaigning for re-election, and sought to deflect blame from himself to China and especially to the WHO for failing to investigate the Chinese origins of the virus and to effectively warn the world about its dangers. The WHO responded to risk to its reputation by establishing the two inquiries.

Inquiry into the zoonotic origins of COVID-19

The technical inquiry was undertaken by the joint expert team, with scientists nominated by Chinese authorities and by the WHO.

The Chinese spokesperson for the team, Mi Feng, was also the spokesperson for the China National Health Commission. He stressed that the team was a partnership between China and the WHO, and would reach a consensus using the combined expertise of the team (WHO, 2021d).

The team presented their preliminary results at a virtual press conference on 9 February 2021 (WHO, 2021d) and in a report published on 30 March 2021 (WHO, 2021e). The team identified four possible causes of the initial outbreak:

- direct transmission from an animal species such as bats to a human;
- indirect transmission through an intermediary species such as pangolins;
- transmission through the food chain, for example via a frozen product;
- an accident, such as a laboratory-related incident (WHO, 2021d).

The team ruled out the possibility of a laboratory accident. When questioned at the press conference, Peter Embarek, a team member, stated:

> We also, in terms of arguments against, look at the fact that nowhere previously was this particular virus researched or identified or known. There had been no publication, no reports of this virus, of another virus extremely linked or closely linked to this, being worked with in any other laboratory in the world. (WHO, 2021d)

The team agreed that the most likely source of the virus was bats, but indicated that more research was needed to identify the precise route of the transmission. The team did not rule out the possibility that frozen cold-chain products played a role in the transmission of the virus, thus keeping open the possibility that the virus originated outside China (WHO, 2021d and 2021e).

The broader inquiry into the global response to the pandemic

The panel undertaking an inquiry into the global response included scientists and technical experts, but given its broader and more policy oriented remit, its membership was more policy and politics-oriented. The panel was co-chaired by politicians with international standing, Ellen Johnson Sirleaf, former President of Liberia and Helen Clark, former Prime Minister of New Zealand. The autonomy of the co-chairs in selecting panellists and in setting terms of references enabled the panel to claim to be independent and to be able to comment critically on the actions of the WHO and other policy makers.

The panel explicitly stated its intention was 'not to assign blame' (The Independent Panel, 2021, p. 21). The panel report dealt with the origins of the virus in a short paragraph that noted bats were the most likely source, but the intermediate host had still to be identified – referencing the work of the technical scientific inquiry (The Independent Panel, 2021, p. 20).

In its second meeting on 20–21 October 2020, the panel agreed a programme of work with four interconnected themes:

- learning from the past, studying previous outbreaks of infectious disease to assess the extent to which lessons had been learnt;
- reviewing the present, examining how and why COVID-19 became a global pandemic;
- evaluating the impact of COVID-19 on people's health and on health-care systems;
- identify lessons for the future.

The panel identified a number of key factors that explained why COVID-19 spread from a small relatively containable epidemic in Wuhan in December 2019 into a major global pandemic by March 2020:

- A failure of foresight: Despite previous 'near misses', such as SARS in 2003, the 2009 H1N1 flu pandemic and the 2014–16 Ebola epidemic, together with warnings from various national and international agencies and experts, countries were not prepared for 'a new fast-moving pathogen' that was 'transmissible in the absence of symptoms' (The Independent Panel, 2021, p. 15) and caused serious illness.
- A failure to invest in protective systems: While many countries, especially high-income countries in North America and Europe, appeared to be well prepared, in reality many lacked 'solid preparedness plans, core public health capacity and organised multi sectoral coordination with clear commitment from the highest national leadership' (The Independent Panel, 2021, p. 18).
- A slow response to risks posed by COVID-19: In some countries there was a rapid response, with action being taken before there was clear evidence of the transmissibility and lethal nature of the new virus. However, in many countries there was '*delay, hesitation* and *denial* with the net result that an outbreak became an epidemic and an epidemic spread to pandemic proportions' (emphasis in the original, The Independent Panel, 2021, p. 21).
- Warnings from the WHO were disregarded: The WHO first became aware that there was an outbreak of pneumonia of unknown causes in Wuhan on 31 December 2019. It monitored the situation, sending a mission to investigate on 20–21 January 2020. On 30 January, following a personal visit to China and advice from the WHO Emergency Committee, the Director-General declared the outbreak a Public Health Emergency of International Concern (The Independent Panel, 2021, p. 24). Many countries did not respond to this warning, and 'February 2020 was a lost month' (The Independent Panel, 2021, p. 29).
- Excess caution: The WHO was restrained by bureaucratic procedures. Initially, it did not alert countries to the possibility of human transmission as there was no proven evidence for it. However, the panel observed that given the current understanding of respiratory infections, 'there is a case for applying the precautionary principle and assuming that in any outbreak caused by a new pathogen of this type, sustained human-to-human transmission will occur unless the evidence specifically indicates otherwise' (The Independent Panel, 2021, pp 25–6).
- A lack of coordinated responses: Countries with effective central decision making and coordination systems responded most quickly and effectively to COVID-19. Countries that had previous experience of managing

epidemics such as SARS in the western Pacific Rim and Ebola in West Africa tended to be better prepared as they could draw on this experience to 'rapidly establish coordination structures, mobilize surge workforces and engage with communities' (The Independent Panel, 2021, p. 31). Countries with the poorest outcomes were those 'had uncoordinated approaches that devalued science, denied the potential impact of the pandemic, delayed comprehensive action, and allowed distrust to undermine efforts' (The Independent Panel, 2021, p. 33).

- International competition over supplies: In early 2020, as the pandemic developed, so countries competed for resources and 'scrambled to get hold of the equipment, supplies, diagnostic tests, advice, funds and workforce' (The Independent Panel, 2021, p. 32).

The panel observed that one of the major mitigating factors in the pandemic was the major and rapid research and development (R&D) response. In response to the Ebola epidemic in 2016, WHO had identified a new model for R&D response to emerging pathogens and had supported the development of a non-profit organisation, the Coalition of Epidemic Preparedness Innovations (CEPI), to fund basic and clinical research (The Independent Panel, 2021, p. 35). CEPI identified and supported some of the early vaccine developers, including teams at Moderna and Oxford University (The Independent Panel, 2021, pp 35–6).

Did these WHO inquiries have the desired impact?

The technical scientific inquiry

This inquiry was designed to identify the origins of the SARS-CoV-2 virus and to show that it was a natural accident rather than a man-made disaster, in particular that the virus had not been developed and released from a Chinese laboratory.

The team was unable to provide clear and definitive proof. In their report, it was asserted that the virus had probably originated in a bat population and had probably been transmitted to humans through an intermediary host, but it was not possible to identify either the original bat source or the intermediate host.

The credibility of the team was undermined in a number of ways. Peter Daszuk was one of the key spokesman for the team and a strong advocate of the view that the virus could not have originated in the laboratory at the Wuhan Institute for Virology. Other researchers have noted his conflict of interest: Daszuk had obtained funding for the institute and had collaborated with its lead researcher, Shi Zhengli (referred to in the media as Bat Lady). Richard Ebright, a leading molecular biologist, noted this conflict of interest, arguing that the investigations Daszuk had participated in, the WHO inquiry and an earlier one sponsored by *The Lancet*, could not 'be considered credible investigations' (Everington, 2021).

While the scientific consensus was that it is unlikely but not impossible for the virus to have originated in a lab (Maxmen and Mallapaty, 2021), key policy makers did not share this view, most notably Joe Biden, who became US president in January 2021. On 26 May 2021, he announced that he had asked the US intelligence community to prepare within 90 days a definitive report on the origins of COVID-19 and to consider 'whether it emerged from human contact with an infected animal or from a laboratory accident' (The White House, 2021). The consensus of the Intelligence Community (IC) was 'the initial SARS-CoV-2 infection was most likely caused by natural exposure to an animal infected with it or a close progenitor virus' but one agency assessed 'with moderate confidence that the first human infection with SARS-CoV-2 most likely was the result of a laboratory-associated incident, probably involving experimentation, animal handling, or sampling by the Wuhan Institute of Virology. These analysts give weight to the inherently risky nature of work on coronaviruses' (IC, 2021, p. 1)

Biden was effectively dismissing other investigations into the origins of the virus, including the WHO inquiry. While President Trump had been willing to support various conspiracy theories about the pandemic, including the theory it had been released from a Chinese lab, Biden was far more circumspect, so his call for further evidence was particularly damaging for the standing and credibility of the WHO inquiry.

The Independent Panel report

The response to this report was more positive, especially in the scientific community. Peter Gluckman, President of the International Science Council (ISC), a non-governmental organisation representing 40 international scientific unions and associations and over 140 national and regional scientific organisations, congratulated the panel on 'its comprehensive, balanced and timely review of the global response to COVID-19' (Gluckman, 2021). The ISC welcomed the panel's recognition of 'the extraordinary successes achieved by the scientific community during the pandemic through open collaboration, data sharing, and investment' (Gluckman, 2021). It accepted the panel's view that there had been an uneven response to the pandemic because of a 'lack of global leadership and solidarity', which had undermined the role of multilateral institutions (Gluckman, 2021).

The panel's report also attracted some media coverage. In the UK, the BBC highlighted the panel's judgement that there had been failures both in the WHO and in the global response. It noted that the WHO should have issued warnings earlier; for example, the warning that COVID-19 was a

Public Health Emergency of International Concern could and should have been issued on 22 January and not delayed until 30 January (BBC, 2021b).

It is not clear that the expert inquiry into the source of the pandemic and the Independent Panel investigation into initial management of the pandemic will re-establish confidence in the WHO. The expert committee was unable to provide definitive answers about the source of the virus, its membership was flawed and compromised, and its findings were disregarded by a key funder, the US. The Independent Panel allocated some of the responsibility and blame for the pandemic to the WHO, accusing it of reacting to events and waiting for data rather than anticipated events and predicting how data was likely to change. However, it also pointed the finger at policy makers in high-income countries in the Global North who failed to respond to WHO warnings and to events that were taking place in other countries, such as the lockdown in Wuhan in late January 2020. The lost February was a major factor in the development of the pandemic. However, given the relatively limited media coverage of the panel's report, it is unlikely to substantially shape global opinion and enhance the WHO's reputation.

Comment

Inquiries are a way of neutralising criticism of an organisation's failure to respond effectively to risk. By appointing independent authoritative experts to investigate its actions, an organisation can acknowledge its failures and shortcomings, make amends to those harmed by its actions, demonstrate a willingness to learn lessons and avoid making the same mistakes in the future. It can re-establish its reputation and its legitimacy.

Those appointing inquiries tend to stress their rational role, in terms of identifying why relevant individuals and organisations failed to recognise and mitigate risks and to find ways in which risk could be more effectively identified and managed in the future. However, inquiries also serve a moral and cathartic function: they provide a way for those affected by a disaster to understand its cause and to identify and allocate blame to those who were responsible.

10

Conclusion: risk and the pandemic

Risk: technical rationality and beyond

The COVID-19 pandemic was inextricably linked to risk. As I note in Chapter 1, risk can be used as a technical concept, a means of using evidence from the past to predict and control the future. It provides a way of predicting the incidence of natural events such as epidemics caused by pathogenic microbes. Risk is also shaped by social relationships. One of its key elements, outcomes, acquires meaning because of its social significance, with distinct values attached to different outcomes. Given such values, social actions are shaped by the desire to minimise bad outcomes. In contemporary societies, it is accepted that governments should seek to protect the public by identifying and mitigating risks. The pandemic provides an opportunity to consider the ways in which governments seek to do this, and the relative success and failure of their choices,

The challenge of dealing with a novel disease

In early 2020, SARS-CoV-2 was a novel virus, and therefore it was difficult to use traditional public health techniques based on epidemiology to predict its impact and to plan responses; there was no evidence on which to base risk assessments. At the start of the pandemic, policy makers had to find a way of making sense of the threat posed by COVID-19. They framed the new disease in different ways, and these frames had important impact on the way in which COVID-19 spread from a localised outbreak in Wuhan into a global pandemic, which within two years had infected over 435 million people and killed nearly 6 million (Johns Hopkins University, 2022).

Framing COVID-19 as a highly infectious lethal disease such as SARS or Ebola

Countries with previous experience of outbreaks of rapidly spreading and highly lethal diseases such as SARS or Ebola mostly framed the new virus in those terms, as a highly infectious and lethal virus, but one that could be identified and controlled using strict public health measures such as travel restrictions, quarantine and track and isolate.

Countries that framed COVID-19 as SARS initially managed the disease effectively, mostly limiting its spread to sporadic cases or small clusters. Taiwan responded rapidly to the first signs of danger, while New Zealand and Senegal used the initial 'quiet' phase in January and February 2020 to plan, so that when the first cases were identified, suggesting community transmission, they were able to adopt public health measures while the numbers were still low. In the first 18 months of the pandemic, Taiwan and New Zealand were virtually COVID-free.

However, there were important differences between SARS and SARS-CoV-2. Generally, SARS was transmitted by symptomatic individuals when the illness was well established, which simplified the task of identifying cases and tracing and isolating contacts. SARS-CoV-2 could be transmitted by individuals who did not have obvious symptoms. This made quarantining and tracking and tracing challenging. In countries that took strong border controls to prevent the entry of the virus, new cases appeared. In New Zealand, 'smouldering transmission' between asymptomatic individuals may explain why new cases were identified after a gap of over 100 days (Wood, 2020).

As the pandemic entered its third year, countries that had adopted a strong public health approach and aimed for a zero-COVID policy faced new challenges. Given low infection rates, there was limited community immunity and often low take-up of vaccines. In Hong Kong, these factors contributed to rapid spread and a high death rate from the Omicron variant in March 2022. Maintaining controls to prevent the spread of new variants resulted in social and political tensions in some countries. In December 2022, public disorder in China forced the Chinese Communist party to relax its strict zero-COVID policy, making it the last country to accept that zero-COVID was unachievable (Mao, 2022).

Framing COVID-19 as seasonal flu

Seasonal flu is a regular occurrence in many countries. While major outbreaks of new variants are relatively uncommon, they do occur, and these countries have well-developed contingency strategies to deal with such outbreaks.

Seasonal flu is difficult to control but, apart from vulnerable individuals, most people have a rather mild and short-lived illness. The harmful effects of flu can be minimised by protecting the most vulnerable individuals in the population by vaccination and/or 'cocooning' – advising these individuals to limit their social contacts. The virus can then be allowed to spread through the rest of the population, and should eventually disappear as the healthy population builds up collective or herd immunity. In most of Europe and the Americas, countries disregarded the initial warning signs in January and February, adopting a wait and see policy and allowing the virus to spread, while mitigating its affect by advising vulnerable individuals to limit their social contacts. However, as community transmission became established, admissions to hospitals and ICUs rose, threatening to overwhelm capacity and staffing. This was followed by increasing death rates, especially among the most vulnerable sections of society. This left policy makers with a difficult choice between a high death rate and a lockdown of economic and social activity. Most chose lockdown.

The rapid development and approval of COVID-19 vaccines in late 2020 provided policy makers in these countries with a way of protecting their populations through mass vaccination programmes. Infection rates remained high in early 2022 and the new dominant variant, Omicron, was more contagious than the variants it replaced but less lethal. Policy makers were able to reduce protective measures and to claim success in containing the pandemic.

Managing risk during the pandemic: probability, outcomes and values

When risk is used to predict the future, it involves the calculation of the probability of one or more outcomes. Most attention is given to harmful outcomes, such as being infected and dying from a lethal virus.

In the early stages of the pandemic, modellers used mathematical models to predict the rate at which the virus was likely to spread and the harm it was likely to cause. Their predictions attracted the attention of policy makers and the mass media, and they contributed to major shifts in policy from herd immunity to lockdown in the UK and US at the end of March 2020, when policy makers realised that the predicted body count was going to be unacceptable.

Things get more complicated and choices more difficult when the outcome is different for different groups or when there are different types of (adverse) outcomes for a specific group, all of which need to be traded off against each other.

Triaging during the peak of the first wave

Triaging is a risk-based decision-making system. It is based on a value system that prioritises the saving of lives. As this value system is widely accepted in modern societies, it tends to be taken for granted. However, using triaging in the pandemic was problematic. Since SARS-CoV-2 caused more serious illness among older people, triaging, while increasing survival rates and enabling doctors and other staff to concentrate their attention on patients who were most likely to survive, effectively denied many older people the intensive care that would maximise their chances of recovery. As I note in Chapter 3, when English newspapers published information about a proposed triaging system, policy makers rapidly distanced themselves from it. While it was acceptable for doctors to use this system informally, it was not acceptable for policy makers to formally acknowledge this and to publicly debate the relative benefit and values of different outcomes.

Risk categorisation

As the pandemic developed, so many high-income countries categorised their populations into COVID-19 risk/disease categories. While whole populations were at risk and required to change their behaviour, there was an emphasis on identifying high-risk groups who were more vulnerable to the virus than other groups and who needed to take extra precautions to protect themselves. The high-risk categorisation of most groups was based on epidemiological evidence. As I note in Case Study 2, the initial categorisation of pregnant women as being high risk was not based on evidence but on the precautionary principle of better safe than sorry. Evidence emerged later in the pandemic that pregnant women were indeed at greater risk than their non-pregnant peers, but it is not clear that the high-risk categorisation actually benefited pregnant women. A high-risk categorisation highlights one specific risk or outcome, that of being infected by SARS-CoV-2 and being seriously ill. However, pregnant women face multiple risks, both from their pregnancy and from other sources such isolation and domestic violence. In so far as their high-risk categorisation reduced their access to support and services, such as antenatal care and vaccination, it undermined their capacity to balance and deal with different risks.

Vaccination

Vaccination was one of the major success stories of the pandemic. Many policy makers, especially in northern Europe, have argued that it is possible to 'learn to live with the virus' by mitigating the effects of infections through vaccination. While vaccination programmes in high-income countries involved a major investment of public money and complex logistical programmes, there was minimal public debate about the possible outcomes of such a programme and about which groups should receive it first. In the UK, decisions about priorities were made behind closed doors by a committee of vaccination experts, the JCVI. There was no public engagement. There was explicit recognition that the choices reflected the important value of protecting the most vulnerable and those who provide health and social care for them. However, allocating vaccines to older and vulnerable people delayed vaccination for other groups who had also suffered during the pandemic, such as young people and those from ethnic minority groups. It also downplayed other possible outcomes, such as disrupting transmission of the virus or addressing social inequalities. The JCVI recognised these issues, but effectively dismissed them by focusing on the practical and technical problems of running a vaccination programme. The priorities were justified pragmatically: since older and vulnerable people were offered and had a high take up rate of the seasonal flu vaccines, it was relatively straightforward to give them COVID-19 vaccinations.

Values and choices

When there are multiple possible outcomes, especially when these impact on different social groups in different ways, then the choices are difficult and involve value judgements. Such judgements should be grounded in collective societal values and therefore, in a democratic society, should involve some public engagement.

Policy makers were unwilling to acknowledge that they had or were making value judgements. These judgements were concealed behind the mantra of 'following the science'. When investigators exposed the ways in which value judgements had been made, as in the 'herd immunity' phase in the UK or in the commissioning and use of a decision-making tool that effectively excluded older people from intensive care, policy makers strongly denied they were making value judgements. While behind closed doors decision making could be justified by the complexity and sensitivity of the issues involved and the need to make quick decisions, it did have some consequences, including:

- undermining public trust in decision making;
- opening the space for alternative pandemic narratives;
- creating the space for conspiracy theories.

Public trust and risk communication

Risk communication can be seen as a technical exercise, summarising information about risk in a message and communicating this message with the public. During the pandemic, policy makers attempted to do this as they needed to communicate information about the risks of COVID-19 and how individuals and social groups could reduce these risks.

Policy makers needed to communicate complex scientific and epidemiological concepts in a way that could be understood and accepted by the population, and would result in behavioural changes that limited or stopped the spread of the virus. The information could be and was simplified, being turned into simple slogans such as the Japanese 3Cs or the New Zealand slogans 'Stay home, break the chain of transmission, and save lives' and 'Unite against COVID-19' (Ardern, 2020c).

However, the extent to which the public is willing to accept such messages is shaped by their willingness to trust the source and by their awareness of different competing messages, which in turn is shaped by existing relations of (mis)trust of experts and government agencies, as well as the extent of vulnerability experienced by citizens.

Factors shaping trust

Trust in messages is shaped by perceptions of the source of those messages. The public tends to trust independent experts far more than they do politicians, so in the UK, experts such as the CMO were seen as more authoritative than politicians. However, politicians can overcome intrinsic mistrust by being empathic, appealing to public altruism and creating the sense of a collective endeavour. In the early stages of the pandemic, New Zealand's prime minister, Jacinda Ardern, was able to project calmness and compassion (Johnson, 2020b). Similarly, Japan's prime minister, Shinzo Abe, was able to use the traditional cultural strategy of humility to communicate the public health message.

As Giddens (1991) has observed, in modern societies there has been a rapid expansion of different forms of communication, so that individuals have access to multiple sources that often provide conflicting messages. The lack of a unified authority and mistrust of sources that claim authority is reflected in the ways individuals and social groups choose to hear messages. Thus, responses to public health messages that COVID-19 vaccines are safe were shaped to a large extent by cultural factors. Individuals and groups who did not identify with experts or share their values were less willing to trust expert advice and more willing to accept alternative messages such as vaccines were unnatural and harmful.

Managing risk through health care and science

Modern societies have developed institutions to identify and manage risk through expert knowledge and the application of technology. The COVID-19 pandemic challenged two key institutions, the scientific community and the health-care system. Both initially struggled to respond to the challenge, but over time adjusted.

Mobilising expert knowledge

One of the distinctive features of the COVID-19 pandemic was the speed with which the scientific community mobilised to identify the threat of the new virus and ways in which it risks could be mitigated. While scientists were able to communicate this knowledge effectively to other scientists through their international networks, they were less successful in communicating it to policy makers and through them to the public. There were a number of problems:

- Receptiveness of policy makers, especially politicians: Politicians in many countries were unwilling or unable to heed the warnings. In China at the start of the pandemic, local officials did not want to disrupt a major national holiday and upset national leaders, so they delayed taking action and thus allowed the virus to escape from Wuhan. In Tanzania, the president, who was aware of the scepticism of religious leaders, denied the existence of the virus. In Brazil, the US and UK, populist leaders tried to minimise the dangers, and delayed taking action until it was too late.
- Poor structures and weak links: Countries that had experienced major outbreaks of infectious disease had often learnt from this experience and had set up national centres to monitor new diseases and plan responses. Taiwan, which had experienced SARS, and Senegal, which was near the West African Ebola outbreak, had both developed national centres that worked closely with policy makers and were therefore able to alert them to the emerging risk of COVID-19. In the US and UK, there were extensive and well-developed scientific communities, but links with the policy community were poorly developed. At the start of the pandemic, the US president had to rely on his security advisers for assessments of the risks. As the pandemic developed, he established and used a task force that included prominent scientists. However, in his desire to control the message, the president marginalised them, disregarding their advice and creating mixed messages.
- Policy makers failed to critically evaluate the advice they were receiving, relying on a small group of expert advisers: During the pandemic, these advisors tended to be established authorities in the medical profession whose advice reflected the dominant consensus. The failure to consider alternative voices can be seen in the droplet versus aerosol debate (see Case Study 6). In Japan, there was collaboration between scientists from different disciplines at the start of the pandemic, and they identified the importance of aerosol spray in the transmission of SARS-CoV-2, contributing to the early adoption of the Japanese 3C policy that stressed the importance of ventilation and mask wearing. In most other countries, infectious disease control specialists played a key role in identifying how the virus was transmitted. These specialists were experts in wound management, and they highlighted the role of larger particles in transmission as well as hygiene measures such as hand washing and disinfecting surfaces in preventing transmission. Policy makers outside Japan initially accepted this advice and downplayed the role of aerosol transmission. It was nearly a year before the scientific consensus shifted

and the importance of aerosol transmission and of ventilation and mask wearing was generally accepted.

It is one of the unfortunate paradoxes of the COVID-19 pandemic that the knowledge necessary to control the spread of the virus was available at an early stage, and if used effectively would have prevented the spread of the virus. Risk assessment is a way of making predictions about the future, and thus it can form the basis of rational decision making – but only if decision makers are able to access and are willing to use this knowledge.

Impact on the health-care system and health-care workers

In modern high-income countries, health-care systems are the main mechanism for identifying and managing the dangers of serious illness. This creates fateful moments that puncture the protective cocoon of normal life and undermine ontological security, the sense that life will carry on as before (Giddens, 1991). Serious illness threatens the very existence of life. The health-care system provides protection and a mechanism for converting the uncertainties of illness into manageable risks and providing hope of a return to pre-illness normality.

For the patient, serious illness is an unexpected, disruptive and often unfamiliar event outside their normal experience. For doctors and nurses working in the health-care system, serious illness is a routine event. While there may be uncertainties about the precise nature of an illness and how it will develop, health professionals have established routines for minimising and managing such uncertainties. These routines not only enable health professionals to make sense of and manage illnesses but they also provide them with a degree of protection against the physical and emotional hazards of caring for and treating people with serious illnesses.

The COVID-19 pandemic undermined health-care systems and disrupted normal routines, increasing uncertainties and exposing health-care staff to new risks and anxieties. At the start of the pandemic, the rapid spread of the virus in countries that adopted a wait and see policy resulted in a swift rise in the number of seriously ill patients, which threatened to overwhelm hospitals. This changed the normal relationship between the health-care system and society, with individuals in countries such as the UK being exhorted to minimise their use of health care.

In health-care systems, the routines that structured everyday activities were disrupted. Health-care staff were faced with uncertainties that were difficult to resolve, a sudden influx of patients with a highly infectious disease that they did not know how to treat and that could infect them, and through them their families and friends. Given the limited resources available, especially ventilators and ICU beds, they had to make difficult decisions about which patients to treat and which to leave to die. In high-income countries, most health systems responded rapidly by moving as many services as possible online, by cancelling all or most non-emergency admissions, by internally dividing space and separating the treatment of COVID-19 and non-COVID-19 patients, and by reallocating staff to the care and treatment of COVID-19 patients. Such measures combined with lockdowns meant that most health-care systems were not overwhelmed and were able to keep functioning.

PPE provided protection for front-line staff. However, in the first wave of the pandemic, most health-care systems were ill-prepared and supplies of PPE did not match the demand. Supplies were restricted to staff working in the most high-risk settings such as ICUs, leaving staff in lower risk areas, for example caring for COVID-19 patients on general wards or in care homes, unprotected. As supplies increased, so did the level of protection, but wearing PPE, especially full body protection, emphasised the dangers of COVID-19 and interfered with key aspects of patient care. It became difficult to communicate with patients and to establish the face-to-face relationships that are essential for personalising an abstract system and for building trust.

COVID-19 disrupted the normal routines of front-line staff in health and social care, breaking the protective cocoon such routines provided. Front-line workers were exposed to the risk of serious illness. The difficulty and emotional stress of managing these risks, for example caring for dying patients, working long hours in unfamiliar roles or avoiding contact with family and friends, are prominent themes in their pandemic narratives.

Moving beyond the technical use of risk: making sense of different realities

Pandemic narratives

Narratives play a key role in making sense of experiences and defining reality. In the COVID-19 pandemic, there were multiple competing narratives that defined the reality and risks of COVID-19 in different ways.

Government narratives focused on numbers, using numbers of cases, hospital admissions and deaths to define the current situation, and the changing pattern of these numbers to predict the future spread of the virus and the need for public health measures such as lockdowns. Government representatives in the UK attached special importance to the R_o, the average number of individuals that one infected person infected. When R_o was above one, the number of cases was rising. However, R_o can only be calculated in retrospect from actual changes in case numbers, and it is based on an average, so the apparent precision of such numbers conceals various assumptions. judgements and time delays. This did not stop ministers and their advisers from using it as a key indicator to justify changing policy.

The focus on numbers tended to block out individual experiences of the pandemic, especially the suffering and injustice it engendered. Such individual stories broke through occasionally in government narratives, but usually this took the form of 'good news' stories such as Captain Tom, who raised substantial sums of money for the NHS.

Government narratives played an important role in shaping public perceptions of the realities and dangers of the COVID-19 pandemic. The media reporting of the pandemic included these facts; however, in much reporting there were narratives in which the facts were combined with and illustrated by personal stories. Such narrative matrices provided an emotional and moral context for the pandemic, enabling the audience to grasp the scale and suffering, and also to identify the failings that contributed to such suffering. Alternative mass media narratives tended to focus on the injustice of the pandemic. The starting point for these could be numbers, for example the number of front-line workers or individuals from ethnic minority groups being infected and dying. The narratives tended to focus on individuals' stories and to highlight the vulnerability of individuals involved and the injustice resulting from failures to identify and mitigate the risks to which they were exposed.

Media narratives drew on individuals' stories, especially those told by survivors of COVID-19 or relatives of those who died. These individuals also used social media and books to tell their stories. Some of these narratives were written by front-line workers, and these provide accounts both of suffering experienced by those that care and those who are treated, and their own struggles to survive.

Alternative versions of reality and risk: conspiracy theories

A feature of the COVID-19 pandemic was the speed with which scientists identified the virus causing the illness, SARS-CoV-2. By March 2020, there was clear evidence of the risks that the virus presented. Paradoxically, this scientific assessment of the risk was almost immediately contested by conspiracy theorists, who either claimed the virus was a product of technology or was a hoax.

Conspiracy theorists such as anti-vaxxers argued that science created and did not mitigate risk. They used pseudo-science to argue that vaccination created risks by introducing foreign and dangerous substances into the body. The pandemic provided ideal conditions for conspiracy theorists. It created fear and anxiety, compounded in some countries by inconsistent public health messaging. The lockdown deprived many people of their normal social networks that would anchor them in shared reality, and this gave them the time and opportunity to surf the internet looking for the 'truth' about COVID-19. Conspiracy theorists were happy to supply their version of the truth, despite the efforts of social media platforms such as Facebook to counter such alternative realities.

Inquiries and hindsight: analysing the failure to identify and prevent risk

As Mary Douglas (1990) has observed, risk, like sin, works backwards as well as forwards. With hindsight, it is possible to unsettle the past and imagine an alternative one. This can be done through an inquiry that asks if things had been done differently and risks properly assessed whether the outcome would have been different.

Some policy makers have argued that a proper inquiry cannot take place until the pandemic is over. This has not stopped inquiries taking place. It has already become clear that in countries with high infection and death rates, such as the US, UK and Brazil, inquiries have blamed policy makers for failing to recognise the risks of SARS-CoV-2 and for failing to take and communicate timely action.

Final comment

In modern society, evaluating risk is a way of managing uncertainty; it provides a way of predicting and controlling the future and accounting for past misfortune. When risk is expressed in numbers, for instance the probability of infections or the number of avoidable deaths, it can be mistaken for objective facts. However, risk is socially constructed and used by individuals and groups to achieve certain objectives. When the survivors of a disasters or relatives of the dead assert the event was not an accident and that individuals and organisations failed to identify and manage the risks, they are seeking to hold those individuals and organisations to account, and to ensure they are punished for their failure.

The emergence of a new highly infectious and lethal virus from Wuhan in late 2019 created uncertainty, and policy makers sought to assess the risk it presented. They constructed this risk in different ways. Those countries that framed it as SARS- or Ebola-like emphasised its lethal aspects, and through zero-COVID policies proactively sought to control the virus. Those countries that framed it as flu-like emphasised its transmissibility, and accepted it was impossible to prevent transmission; they initially adopted wait and see policies while warning vulnerable individuals to protect themselves.

It is possible to argue that given the limited information available at the time, policy makers did the best they could, and that with the benefit of hindsight it is possible to see that they could have done better. It will be interesting to see whether history will be so kind and forgiving.

References

Aamir, A. (2020) 'Conspiracy theories help coronavirus take root in Pakistan', NIKKEI Asia, 13 June, Available from: https://asia.nikkei.com/Spotlight/Coronavirus/Conspiracy-theories-help-coronavirus-take-root-in-Pakistan [Accessed 2 September 2022].

Abutaleb, Y and Plaletta, D. (2021) *Nightmare Scenario: Inside the Trump Administration's Response to the Pandemic that Changed History*, New York, HarperCollins.

Africa CDC (2021a) 'About Us', Africa CDC, Available from: https://africacdc.org/about-us/ [Accessed 12 October 2021].

Africa CDC (2021b) 'Research and Development Priorities for COVID-19 in Africa', Africa CDC, February, Available from: https://ajph.aphapublications.org/doi/full/10.2105/AJPH.93.3.383 [Accessed 12 October 2021].

Ahluwalia, S.C., Edelen, M.O., Qureshi, N. and Etchegaray, J.M. (2021) 'Trust in experts, not trust in national leadership, leads to greater uptake of recommended actions during the COVID-19 pandemic', *Risk, Hazards and Crisis in Public Policy*, 12(3): 283–302.

Alaszewska, J. and Alaszewski, A. (2015) 'Purity and danger: shamans, diviners and the control of danger in premodern Japan as evidenced by the healing rites of the Aogashima islanders', *Health, Risk & Society*, 17(3–4): 302–25.

Alaszewski, A. (2003) 'Risk, trust and health', *Health, Risk & Society*, 5(3): 235–9.

Alaszewski, A. (2015) 'Anthropology and risk: insights into uncertainty, danger and blame from other cultures – a review essay', *Health, Risk & Society*, 17(3–4): 205–25.

Alaszewski, A. (2020) 'Should pregnant women be in a high risk Covid-19 category?' *British Journal of Midwifery*, 28(10): 732–4.

Alaszewski, A. (2021a) *COVID-19 and Risk: Policy Making in a Global Pandemic*, Bristol: Policy Press.

Alaszewski, M. (2021b) To jab or not to jab? Covid vaccination dilemmas, *Law Society Gazette*, 27 September, Available from: https://www.lawgazette.co.uk/legal-updates/to-jab-or-not-to-jab-covid-vaccination-dilemmas/5109888.article [Accessed 30 September 2021].

Alaszewski, A. and Brown, P. (2007) 'Risk, uncertainty and knowledge', *Health, Risk & Society*, 9(1): 1–10.

Alaszewski, A. and Brown, P. (2012) *Making Health Policy: A Critical Introduction*, Cambridge: Polity Press.

Alaszewski, A. and Horlick-Jones, T. (2003) 'How can doctors communicate about risk more effectively?' *BMJ*, 327(7417): 728–31, Available from: doi:10.1136/bmj.327.7417.728 [Accessed 20 August 2022].

Álvares, D. and Jeanet, D. (2021) 'Senate report urges charging Brazil's leader over pandemic', AP News, 20 October, Available from: https://apnews.com/article/coronavirus-pandemic-crime-pandemics-homicide-covid-19-pandemic-1a1f8bf555e837c16dcfeaec111a7d3e [Accessed 29 January 2021].

Andrade, G. (2020) 'Medical conspiracy theories: cognitive science and implications for ethics', *Medicine, Health Care and Philosophy*, 2020, 16 April, p. 1–14, Available from: https://www.ncbi.nlm.nih.gov/pmc/articles/PMC7161434/#CR28 [Accessed 20 August 2022].

Andrade, G.E. and Hussain, A. (2018) 'Polio in Pakistan: political, sociological, and epidemiological factors', *Cureus*, 10(10), Available from: https://www.ncbi.nlm.nih.gov/pmc/articles/PMC6318131/ [Accessed 20 August 2022].

Aptaclub (2020) 'Over half of pregnant women and new mums feel anxious or lonely during ongoing Covid crisis', press release, 22 June.

Aronowitz, R.A. (2008) 'Framing disease: an under appreciated mechanism for the social patterning of health', *Social Science & Medicine*, 67: 1–9.

Aronowitz, R.A. (2009) 'The converged experience of risk and disease', *The Milbank Quarterly*, 87 (2): 417–42.

Ardern, J. (2020a) 'Prime minister: COVID-19 alert level increased', 23 March, Available from: www.beehive.govt.nz/speech/prime-minister-covid-19-alert-level-increased [Accessed 15 December 2020].

Ardern, J. (2020b) 'Review of COVID-19 Alert Level 2', Available from: https://covid19.govt.nz/assets/resources/proactive-release-2020-july/AL2-Minute-and-Paper-CAB-20-MIN-0270-Review-of-COVID-19-Alert-Level-2-8-June-2020.pdf [Accessed 15 December 2020].

Ardern, J. (2020c) '"Stay at home, break the chain, and save lives": NZ PM', 27 March, Available from: www.news.com.au/world/stay-at-home-break-the-chain-and-save-lives-nz-pm/ video/45a684a63759808d9a2b4ef4f240ed24 [Accessed 15 December 2020].

Armstrong, D. (1995) 'The rise of surveillance medicine', *Sociology of Health and Illness*, 17 (3): 393–404.

Armstrong-Hough, M.J. (2015) 'Performing prevention: risk, responsibility, and reorganising the future in Japan during the H1N1 pandemic', *Health, Risk & Society*, 17(3–4): 285–301.

Ashworth, E. (2020) 'Covid-19 and the UK's maternity services', Available from: www.aims.org.uk/journal/item/giving-birth-in-covid-19 [Accessed 6 July 2020].

Associated Press (2022) 'Protests against Covid restrictions held in France and Netherlands', *The Guardian*, 12 February, Available from: https://www.theguardian.com/world/2022/feb/12/covid-pass-protesters-convoy-paris-police.

Audet, C. (2020) 'Giving birth amid a pandemic in Belgium: the challenges faced by mothers and midwives', Available from: https://blogs.bmj.com/covid-19/2020/04/30/giving-birth-amid-a-pandemic-in-belgium-the-challenges-faced-by-mothers-and-midwives/ [Accessed 4 September 2020].

Bariyo, N. (2021) 'Tanzania's new president nudges country away from Covid-19 denial', *Wall Street Journal*, 12 April, Available from: https://www.wsj.com/articles/tanzanias-president-nudges-country-away-from-covid-19-denial-11618247113 [Accessed 14 April 2021].

Barnes, O. and Neville, S. (2022) 'NHS trusts in England declare critical incident as hospital admissions near January high', *Financial Times*, 7 April, Available from: https://www.ft.com/content/8dbb5830-768a-4eae-93a1-a03f9b7dc87f [Accessed 8 April 2022].

Barr, C., Kommenda, N., McIntyre, N. and Voce, A. (2020a) 'Revealed: scale of coronavirus's deadly toll of ethnic minorities', *The Guardian*, 23 April.

Barr, C., Kommenda, N., McIntyre, N. and Voce, A. (2020b) 'Ethnic minorities dying of Covid-19 at higher rate, analysis shows', *The Guardian*, 23 April, Available from: https://www.theguardian.com/world/2020/apr/22/racial-inequality-in-britain-found-a-risk-factor-for-covid-19 [Accessed 5 December 2022].

BBC (1999) 'Ward known as "departure lounge"', BBC News, 19 October, Available from: http://news.bbc.co.uk/1/hi/health/background_briefings/the_bristol_heart_babies/478560.stm [Accessed 17 April 2022].

BBC (2020a) 'Coronavirus: New Zealand minister resigns after lock-down blunders', BBC News, 2 July, Available from: www.bbc.co.uk/news/world-asia-53259236 [Accessed 15 December 2020].

BBC (2020b) 'The forgotten frontline', *Panorama*, BBC, 30 July, Available from: www.bbc.co.uk/programmes/m000lbq0 [Accessed 15 December 2020].

BBC (2020c) 'Coronavirus: UK tactics defended as cases expected to rise', BBC News, 10 March, Available from: https://www.bbc.co.uk/news/uk-51812326 [Accessed 2 November 2021].

BBC (2020d) 'Coronavirus: WHO advises to wear masks in public areas', BBC News, 6 June, Available from: www.bbc.co.uk/news/health-52945210 [Accessed 15 December 2020].

BBC (2020e) '"We didn't have exact measures" in place for Covid says ex-civil service head', BBC News, 21 October, Available from: www.bbc.co.uk/news/uk-politics-54617148 [Accessed 15 December 2020].

BBC (2020f) 'Ischgl: Austria sued over Tyrol ski resort's Covid-19 out-break', BBC News, 23 September, Available from: www.bbc.co.uk/news/world-europe-54256463 [Accessed 15 December 2020].

BBC (2020g) 'Coronavirus: Prof Neil Ferguson quits government role after "undermining" lockdown', BBC News, 6 May, Available from: https://www.bbc.co.uk/news/uk-politics-52553229 [Accessed 3 November 2021].

BBC (2020h) 'Coronavirus: The world in lockdown in maps and charts', BBC News, 7 April, Available from: https://www.bbc.co.uk/news/world-52103747 [Accessed 21 June 2022].

BBC (2021a) 'Covid: Boris Johnson resisted autumn lockdown as only over-80s dying – Dominic Cummings', BBC News, 20 July, Available from: https://www.bbc.co.uk/news/uk-politics-57854811 [Accessed 20 July 2021].

BBC (2021b) 'Covid: serious failures in WHO and global response, report finds', BBC News, 12 May, Available from: https://www.bbc.co.uk/news/world-57085505 [Accessed 10 July 2021].

BCNU (2021) 'BCCDC now recognizes airborne transmission of COVID-19', BCNU, 8 January, Available from: https://www.bcnu.org/News-Eve nts/Pages/BCCDC-Now-Recognizes-Airborne-Transmission.aspx [30 November 2021].

Beck, U. (1992) *Risk Society: Towards a New Modernity*, London and Thousand Oaks, CA: Sage.

Bernstein, P.L. (1996) *Against the Gods: The Remarkable Story of Risk*, New York: John Wiley and Sons.

Birmingham City University (2020) 'COVID-19 sparks online Islamophobia as fake news and racist memes are shared online, new research finds, Birmingham City University', Available from: https://www.bcu.ac.uk/about-us/coronavirus-information/news/covid-19-sparks-online-islam ophobia-as-fake-news-and-racist-memes-are-shared-online-new-resea rch-finds [Accessed 2 September 2022].

Bjorklund, K. and Ewing, A. (2020) 'The Swedish COVID-19 response is a disaster: it shouldn't be a model for the rest of the world', *Time*, 14 October, Available from: https://time.com/5899432/sweden-coronovi rus-disaster/ [Accessed 14 September 2022].

Bourdieu, P. (1977) *Outline of a Theory of Practice*, Cambridge: Cambridge University Press.

BRI Inquiry (2001) *Learning from Bristol: The Report of the Public Inquiry into Children's Heart Surgery at the Bristol Royal Infirmary 1984–1995*, Chair Ian Kennedy, CM 5207, London: HMSO, Available from: https://webarch ive.nationalarchives.gov.uk/20090811154614/http://www.bristol-inquiry. org.uk/final_report/report/Summary4.htm [Accessed 14 October 2020].

Brown, P. and Calnan, M. (2012) *Trusting on the Edge: Managing Uncertainty and Vulnerability in the midst of Mental Health Problems*, Bristol: Policy Press.

Brown, P. and Levinson, S.C. (1987) *Politeness: Some Universals in Language Usage*, Cambridge: Cambridge University Press.

BMJ (2019) 'Richard Lacey: microbiologist who came under fire for claiming a link between mad cow disease and variant CJD in humans', *BMJ*, 364, Available from: https://doi.org/10.1136/bmj.l1078 [Accessed 1 March 2021].

BSE Inquiry (2000) *The Report, Findings and Conclusions*, vol 1, Chair: Lord Phillips, Available from: https://webarchive.nationalarchives.gov.uk/200 60308232515/http://www.bseinquiry.gov.uk/pdf/index.htm [Accessed 19 July 2021].

Burgess, A. (2002) 'Comparing national responses to perceived health risks from mobile phone masts', *Health, Risk & Society*, 4(2): 175–88.

Burgess A. (2017) 'The development of risk politics in the UK: Thatcher's "remarkable" but forgotten "don't die of ignorance" AIDS campaign', *Health, Risk & Society*, 19(5–6): 227–45.

Burgess, A. and Horii, M. (2012) 'Risk, ritual and health responsibilisation: Japan's "safety blanket" of surgical mask wearing', *Sociology of Health & Illness*, 34(8): 1184–98.

Cabinet Office (2020) 'Staying alert and safe (social distancing)', 11 May, Available from: www.gov.uk/government/publications/staying-alert-and-safe-social-distancing/staying-alert-and-safe-social-distancing [Accessed 18 May 2020].

California Department of Public Health (2021) 'Cases and deaths associated with COVID-19 by age group in California, 8 September 2021', Available from: https://www.cdph.ca.gov/Programs/CID/DCDC/Pages/COVID-19/COVID-19-Cases-by-Age-Group.aspx [Accessed 13 September 2021].

Calvert, J. and Arbuthnott, G. (2021) *Failures of State: The Inside Story of Britain's Battle with Coronavirus*, London: Mudlark.

Campbell, A. (2006a) *Spring of Fear*, Chapter 1, The Sars Commission, Available from: www.archives.gov.on.ca/en/e_records/sars/report/v2-pdf/Vol2Chp1.pdf [Accessed 15 December 2020].

Campbell, A. (2006b) *Spring of Fear*, Chapter 9: Recommendations, The Sars Commission, Available from: www.archives.gov.on.ca/en/e_records/sars/report/v3-pdf/Vol3Chp9.pdf [Accessed 15 December 2020].

Campbell, D., Topping, A. and Barr, C. (2020) 'Virus patients more likely to die may have ventilators taken away', *The Guardian*, 1 April, Available from: www.theguardian.com/society/2020/apr/01/ventilators-may-be-taken-from-stable-coronavirus-patients-for-healthier-ones-bma-says [Accessed 15 December 2020].

Camus, A. (1960) *The Plague*, Harmondsworth: Penguin.

Canadian Institute for Health Information (2021) 'The impact of COVID-19 on long-term care in Canada: focus on the first 6 months', Ottawa, ON: CIHI, Available from: https://www.cihi.ca/sites/default/files/docum ent/impact-covid-19-long-term-care-canada-first-6-months-report-en.pdf [Accessed 14 September 2021].

CARE (2020) 'Vaccins contre le SARS-CoV-2: Une Strategie de Vaccination', 9 July, Available from: www.scribd.com/document/470275 663/avis-vaccins-9-juillet-2020-care-conseil-scientifique-comite-vaccin-pdf#fullscreen&from_embed [Accessed 15 December 2020].

Carter, H. (2020) 'MMR scandal doctor Andrew Wakefield now claiming coronavirus is a HOAX in new anti-vaccine campaign', *The Sun*, 17 July, Available from: https://www.thesun.co.uk/news/12149075/andrew-wakefield-claiming-coronavirus-is-a-hoax/ [Accessed 14 September 2021].

Caserotti, M., Girardi, P., Rubaltelli, E., Tasso, A. Lotto, L and Gavaruzzi, T. (2021) 'Associations of COVID-19 risk perception with vaccine hesitancy over time for Italian residents', *Social Science and Medicine*, 272(113688): 1–9.

Cathey, L. (2020) '5 mixed messages from Trump that have marred his administration's coronavirus response', ABC News, 19 March, Available from: https://abcnews.go.com/Politics/mixed-messages-trump-marred-administrations-coronavirus-response/story?id=69625769 [Accessed 6 April 2022].

CDC (2007) 'Guideline for isolation precautions: preventing transmission of infectious agents in healthcare settings', Available from: https://www.cdc.gov/infectioncontrol/guidelines/isolation/index.html [Accessed 11 March 2021].

CDC (2014) 'Guidance on Personal Protective Equipment (PPE) to be used by healthcare workers during management of patients with confirmed Ebola or persons under investigation (PUIs) for Ebola who are clinically unstable or have bleeding, vomiting, or diarrhea in U.S. hospitals, including procedures for donning and doffing PPE', Available from: https://www.cdc.gov/vhf/ebola/healthcare-us/ppe/guidance.html [Accessed 11 March 2021].

CDC (2020a) 'Coronavirus disease 2019 (Covid-19): people who are at higher risk for severe illness', Available from: www.cdc.gov/coronavirus/2019-ncov/need-extra-precautions/people-at-higher-risk.html [Accessed 14 May 2020].

CDC (2020b) 'Considerations for wearing masks', updated 4 November, Available from: www.cdc.gov/coronavirus/2019-ncov/prevent-getting-sick/cloth-face-cover-guidance.html [Accessed 15 December 2020].

CDC (2020c) 'Impact of the COVID-19 pandemic on emergency department visits – United States, January 1, 2019–May 30, 2020', *Morbidity and Mortality Reports*, 12 June, 69(23): 699–704, Available from: https://www.cdc.gov/mmwr/volumes/69/wr/mm6923e1.htm [Accessed 8 March 2021].

CDC (2020d) 'CDC calls on Americans to wear masks to prevent COVID-19 spread', CDC Newsroom, 14 July, Available from: https://www.cdc.gov/media/releases/2020/p0714-americans-to-wear-masks.html [Accessed 28 October 2021].

CDC (2021a) 'Similarities and differences between flu and COVID-19', CDC, Available from: https://www.cdc.gov/flu/symptoms/flu-vs-covid19.htm [Accessed 26 August 2021].

CDC (2021b) 'Pregnant and recently pregnant people: at increased risk for severe illness from COVID-19', Available from: https://www.cdc.gov/coronavirus/2019-ncov/need-extra-precautions/pregnant-people.html [Accessed 16 September 2021].

CDC (2021c) 'Role of the Advisory Committee on Immunization Practices in CDC's vaccine recommendations', Available from: https://www.cdc.gov/vaccines/acip/committee/role-vaccine-recommendations.html [Accessed 20 September 2021].

CDC (2021d) 'Benefits of getting a COVID-19 vaccine', CDC, Updated 16 August 2021, Available from: https://www.cdc.gov/coronavirus/2019-ncov/vaccines/vaccine-benefits.html [Accessed 28 September 2021].

CDC (2021e) 'Interim infection prevention and control recommendations for healthcare personnel during the coronavirus disease 2019 (COVID-19) pandemic', 23 February, Available from: https://www.cdc.gov/coronavirus/2019-ncov/hcp/infection-control-recommendations.html [Accessed 21 March 2021].

CDC (2021f) 'Guidance for wearing masks: help slow the spread of COVID-19', updated 19 April, Available from: https://www.cdc.gov/coronavirus/2019-ncov/prevent-getting-sick/cloth-face-cover-guidance.htm [Accessed 17 January 2022].

CDC (2022a) 'Vaccine basics', 8 August, Available from: https://www.cdc.gov/smallpox/vaccine-basics/index.html [Accessed 5 September 2022].

CDC (2022b) 'Overview of COVID-19 vaccines', 2 September, Available from: https://www.cdc.gov/coronavirus/2019-ncov/vaccines/different-vaccines/overview-COVID-19-vaccines.html [Accessed 5 September 2022].

Central People's Government of the People's Republic of China (2020) 'COVID-19 vaccine development, priority populations and pricing', press release, 20 October, Available from: http://www.gov.cn/fuwu/2020-10/20/content_5552857.htm [Accessed 20 September 2020].

Cepelewicz, J (2021) 'The hard lessons of modeling the coronavirus pandemic', *Quanta Magazine*, 28 January, Available from: https://www.quantamagazine.org/the-hard-lessons-of-modeling-the-coronavirus-pandemic-20210128/ [Accessed 25 August 2021].

Chen, L. (2020) 'The US has a lot to learn from Taiwan's Covid fight', *CNN Opinion*, 10 July, Available from: https://edition.cnn.com/2020/07/10/opinions/taiwan-covid-19-lesson-united-states-chen/index.html [Accessed 15 December 2020].

Chivers, T. (2022) 'How Hong Kong went from Zero Covid success story to the world's worst Omicron wave', *The Independent,* 15 March, Available from: https://inews.co.uk/news/science/how-hong-kong-went-from-zero-covid-success-story-to-the-worlds-worst-omicron-wave-1517171 [Accessed 24 March 2022].

Claeson, M. and Hanson, S. (2021) 'COVID-19 and the Swedish enigma', *The Lancet*, 397(10271): 259–61, 23 January, Available from: https://www.thelancet.com/article/S0140-6736(20)32750-1/fulltext [Accessed 13 August 2021].

Clarke, R. (2021) *Breathtaking: Inside the NHS in a Time of Pandemic*, London, Little, Brown.

Clarke, A.P., Squire, D. and Bailey, T. (2001) *Marchioness/ Bowbelle: Formal Investigation under the Merchant Shipping Act 1995, Volume I*, London: The Stationery Office, Available from: https:// webarchive.nationalarchives.gov.uk/20141008142557uo_/ http://assets.dft.gov.uk/marchioness-bowbelle.org.uk/report/fi_ report.pdf [Accessed 15 December 2020].

COBR (2021) 'Press conference slides', 22 February, Available from: https://assets.publishing.service.gov.uk/government/uploads/system/uploads/attachment_data/file/963599/2021-02-22_COVID-19_Press_Conference_Slides.pdf [Accessed 24 August 2021].

Cochrane, A. (1972) *Effectiveness and Efficiency: Random Reflections on Health Services*, London: The Nuffield Provincial Hospital Trust, Available from: https://www.nuffieldtrust.org.uk/files/2017-01/effectiveness-and-efficiency-web-final.pdf [Accessed 26 November 2021].

Coderey, C. (2015) 'Coping with health-related uncertainties and risks in Rakhine (Myanmar)', *Health, Risk & Society*, 17(3–4): 263–84.

Cookson, C. (2021) 'Wellcome director resigns as UK government science adviser', *Financial Times*, 2 November.

Corlett, E. (2021) ' "Big questions": New Zealand Covid minister raises doubts about elimination strategy', *The Guardian*, 23 August, Available from: https://www.theguardian.com/world/2021/aug/23/big-questions-new-zealand-covid-minister-raises-doubts-about-elimination-strategy [Accessed 23 August 2021].

Craft, L. (2020) 'Japan has long accepted COVID's airborne spread, and scientists say ventilation is key', CBS News, 13 July, Available from: https://www.cbsnews.com/news/coronavirus-japan-has-long-accepted-covids-airborne-spread-and-scientists-say-ventilation-is-key/ [Accessed 24 November 2021].

Crawford, D.H. (2021) *Viruses – The Invisible Enemy*, Oxford: Oxford University Press.

Crowson, I. and Bennett, A. (2020) 'Virus tragedy: pregnant nurse, 28, dies of coronavirus five days after her baby is saved by emergency C-section in "beacon of light"', *The Sun*, 15 April, Available from: https://www.thesun.co.uk/news/11403855/pregnant-nurse-dies-coronavirus-baby/ [Accessed 1 December 2020].

Cumberland News (2016) 'Thirty years after the Chernobyl disaster', *Cumberland News*, 28 April, Available from: https://www.newsands tar.co.uk/news/16701429.thirty-years-after-the-chernobyl-disaster/ [Accessed 1 July 2022].

Cummings, D. (2021) Twitter, 26 May, Available from: https://twitter.com/Dominic2306/status/1397452170249842691/photo/1 [Accessed 19 August 2021].

Cunningham, S. (2021) 'Unvaxxed? Football could take a leaf out of the NBA book', *The Independent*, 5 October, p. 55.

Daly, R. (2020) 'Ian Brown likens coronavirus to "common cold" in new tweet', *NME*, 18 October, Available from: www.nme.com/news/music/ian-brown-likens-coronavirus-common-cold-new-tweet-2790209 [Accessed 15 December 2020].

Davies, S. (2020) 'Oral evidence: coronavirus: lessons learnt', HC 877, House of Commons, Available from: https://committees.parliament.uk/oralevidence/1323/pdf/ [Accessed 23 August 2021].

Defoe, D. (1722) *A Journal of the Plague Year being Observations or Memorials of the most Remarkable Occurrences as well Publick as Private which happened in London during the last Great Visitation in 1665*, London: E. Nutt.

De Graaff, B., Bal, J., and Bal, R. (2021) 'Layering risk work amidst an emerging crisis: an ethnographic study on the governance of the COVID-19 pandemic in a university hospital in the Netherlands', *Health, Risk and Society*, 23(3–4): 111–27.

De Melo, T. and Figueirdo, C.M.S. (2021) 'Comparing new articles and tweets about COVID-19 in Brazil: Sentiment analysis and topic modelling approach', *JMIR Public Health Surveillance*, 7(2): e24585, Available from: https://www.ncbi.nlm.nih.gov/pmc/articles/PMC7886485/ [Accessed 7 January 2022].

Department of Health (1993) *The Health of the Nation Key Area Handbook: Accidents*, Leeds: Department of Health.

Derosier, J-P. and Toulemonde, G. (2020) *The French Parliament in the Time of Covid-19: Parliament on Life Support*, Paris and Brussels, Foundation Robert Schumann, Available from: https://www.robert-schuman.eu/en/doc/ouvrages/FRS_French_Parliament_Covid-19.pdf [Accessed 31 January 2022].

Dibben, M. R. and Lean, M. (2003) 'Achieving compliance in chronic illness management: illustrations of trust relationships between physicians and nutrition clinic patients', *Health, Risk & Society*, 5(3): 241–58.

Douglas, M. (1966) *Purity and Danger: An Analysis of Concepts of Pollution and Taboo*, London: Routledge and Kegan Paul.

Douglas, M. (1990) 'Risk as a forensic resource', *Daedalus: Journal of the American Academy of Arts and Sciences*, 119(4): 1–16.

Douglas, M. (1992) *Risk and Blame: Essays in Cultural Theory*, London: Routledge.

Douglas, M. and Calvez, M. (1990) 'The self as risk taker: a cultural theory of contagion in relation to AIDS', *Sociological Review*, 38(3): 445–64.

D'Souza, G.A. and Dowdy, D. (2021) 'Rethinking Herd Immunity and the Covid-19 Response End Game', 13 April, Available from: https://publichealth.jhu.edu/2021/what-is-herd-immunity-and-how-can-we-achieve-it-with-covid-19 [Accessed 5 December 2021].

Economist, The (2021) 'Australia is ending its zero-covid strategy: the Delta variant has made it untenable', *The Economist*, 28 August, Available from: https://www.economist.com/asia/2021/08/28/australia-is-ending-its-zero-covid-strategy [Accessed 15 August 2022].

Editors of the Lancet (2004) 'A statement by the editors of the Lancet', Available from: https://www.thelancet.com/pb-assets/Lancet/extras/statement20Feb2004web.pdf [Accessed 25 April 2022].

Ejaz, W., Ittefaq, M., Seo, H. and Naz, F. (2021) 'Factors associated with the belief in COVID-19 related conspiracy theories in Pakistan', *Health, Risk & Society*, 23(3–4): 162–8.

Ekawati, A. (2021) 'Indonesia's COVID vaccination campaign prioritizes workers, 22 January', Available from: https://www.dw.com/en/indonesias-covid-vaccination-campaign-prioritizes-workers/a-56316852 [Accessed 20 September 2021].

El Daif, E. (2021) 'Changing the paradigm of health emergency management, Dalberg', April, https://dalberg.com/our-ideas/interview-with-dr-abdoulaye-bousso-english/ [Accessed 14 October 2021].

Elston, J. W. T., Danis, K., Gray, N. et al (2020) 'Maternal health after Ebola: unmet needs and barriers to healthcare in rural Sierra Leone', *Health Policy and Planning*, 35(1): 78–90, Available from: doi: 10.1093/heapol/czz102 [Accessed 15 December 2020].

Elwell-Sutton, T., Deeny, S. and Stafford, M. (2020) 'Emerging findings on the impact of COVID-19 on black and minority ethnic people', 20 May, Available from: www.health.org.uk/news-and-comment/charts-and-infographics/emerging-findings-on-the-impact-of-covid-19-on-black-and-min [Accessed 15 December 2020].

Everington, K. (2021) 'WHO inspector has conflict of interest in Wuhan COVID probe: Prominent biologist', *Taiwan News*, 2 April, Available from: https://www.taiwannews.com.tw/en/news/4119101 [Accessed 10 July 2021].

Faccin, M., Gargiulo, F., Atlani-Duault, L. and Ward, J.K. (2022) 'Assessing the influence of French vaccine critics during the two first years of the COVID-19 pandemic', *PLoS ONE*, 17(8): Available from: https://journals.plos.org/plosone/article?id=10.1371/journal.pone.0271157 [Accessed 13 September 2022].

Fage-Butler, A. M. (2017) 'Risk resistance: constructing home birth as morally responsible on an online discussion group', *Health, Risk & Society*, 19(3–4): 130–44.

Farrar, J. with Ahuja, A. (2022) *Spike: The Virus vs the People, The Inside Story*, London: Profile Books.

Ferguson, N.M. et al (2020) 'Impact of non-pharmaceutical interventions (NPIs) to reduce COVID-19 mortality and healthcare demand', Imperial College London, 16 March, Available from: www.imperial.ac.uk/media/ imperial-college/medicine/sph/ide/gida-fellowships/Imperial-College-COVID19-NPI-modelling-16-03-2020.pdf [Accessed 15 December 2020].

Fifield, A. (2020) 'In Wuhan's virus wards, plenty of stress but shortages of everything else', *Washington Post*, 24 January, Available from: https:// www.washingtonpost.com/world/asia_pacific/in-wuhans-virus-wards-plenty-of-stress-but-shortages-of-everything-else/2020/01/24/ba1c7 0f0-3ebb-11ea-afe2-090eb37b60b1_story.html [Accessed 9 March 2021].

Financial Times (2020) 'COVID-19 decision support tool', Available from: https://prod-upp-image-read.ft.com/765d3430-7a57-11ea-af44-daa3def9ae03 [Accessed 20 April 2020].

Finucane, M. L., Slovic, P., Mertz, C.K., Flynn, J. and Satterfield, T.A. (2000) 'Gender, race, and perceived risk: the 'white male' effect', *Health, Risk & Society*, 2(2): 159–72.

Foster, P. and Neville, S. (2020) 'How poor planning left the UK without enough PPE', *Financial Times*, 1 May, Available from: https://www.ft.com/ content/9680c20f-7b71-4f65-9bec-0e9554a8e0a7

Foucault, M. (1967) *Madness and Civilization: A History of Insanity in the Age of Reason*, London: Tavistock.

Fox, R.C. (2003) 'Medical uncertainty revisited', in Albrecht, G. L., Fitzpatrick, R. and Scrimshaw, S.C. (eds) *Handbook of Social Studies in Health and Medicine*, London: SAGE, pp 408–25.

Francis, G. (2021) *Intensive Care: A GP, a Community & COVID-19*, London: Profile Books in association with Wellcome Collection.

Frank, D.A., Slovic, P. and Vastfjall, D. (2011) 'Statistics don't bleed': rhetorical psychology, presence, and psychic numbing in genocide pedagogy', *JAC A Journal of Composition Theory*, 31(3/4): 609–24.

Freeman, M. (2020) 'The coronavirus 5G connection and coverup', 18 February, Available from: https://davidicke.com/2020/02/19/coronavi rus-5g-connection-coverup/ [Accessed 15 December 2020].

Full Fact (2020) 'Here is the transcript of what Boris Johnson said on *This Morning* about the new coronavirus', 10 March, Available from: https:// fullfact.org/health/coronavirus/ [Accessed 15 December 2020].

Gabe, M. (2021) 'The critical theory of world risk society: a retrospective analysis', *Risk Analysis*, 41(3): 533–43.

Gallagher, P. (2021) 'Almost 225,000 people waiting over a year for hospital treatment due to Covid-19 effect on the NHS', *inews*, 11 February, Available from: https://inews.co.uk/nhs/number-patients-england-waiting-year-hospital-treatment-highest-since-2008-867566 [Accessed 4 December 2022].

Gerstein, D.M. (2020) 'Assessing the US government response to the coronavirus', *Bulletin of the Atomic Scientists*, 76(4): 166–74, Available from: https://www.tandfonline.com/doi/pdf/10.1080/00963402.2020.1778356?needAccess=true [Accessed 26 October 2021].

Ghebreyesus, T.A. (2020a) 'WHO Director-General's opening remarks at the media briefing on COVID-19 – 11 March 2020', WHO, Available from: www.who.int/dg/speeches/detail/who-director-general-s-opening-remarks-at-the-media-briefing-on-covid-19—11-march-2020 [Accessed 15 December 2020].

Ghebreyesus, T.A. (2020b) 'WHO Director-General's opening remarks at the media briefing on COVID-19 – 5 June 2020', Available from: www.who.int/director-general/speeches/detail/who-director-general-s-opening-remarks-at-the-media-briefing-on-covid-19---5-june-2020 [Accessed 15 December 2020].

Giddens, A. (1990) *The Consequences of Modernity*, Cambridge: Polity Press.

Giddens, A. (1991) *Modernity and Self-Identity: Self and Society in the Late Modern Age*, Cambridge: Polity Press.

Giddens, A. (1999) 'Globalisation', Reith Lectures, Runaway World, BBC Radio 4, Available from: http://downloads.bbc.co.uk/rmhttp/radio4/transcripts/1999_reith1.pdf [Accessed 5 September 2022].

Givon, T. and Young, P. (2001) 'Cooperation and interpersonal manipulation in the society of intimates', in Shibatani, M. (ed.) *The Grammar and Causation of Interpersonal Manipulation*, Amsterdam and Philadelphia: John Benjamins Publishing Company, pp 23–56.

Glezen, W.P., Greenberg, S.B. and Atmar, R.L. (2000) 'Impact of respiratory virus infections on persons with chronic underlying conditions', *JAMA*, 283(4): 499–505, Available from: https://jamanetwork.com/journals/jama/fullarticle/192328 [Accessed 1 September 2021].

Gluckman, P. (2021) 'A response to the Independent Panel for Pandemic Preparedness and Response's new report on the international health response to the COVID-19 pandemic', Available from: https://council.science/current/blog/a-response-to-the-independent-panel-for-pandemic-preparedness-and-responses-new-report-on-the-international-health-response-to-the-covid-19-pandemic/ [10 July 2021].

Goffman, E. (1975) *Frame Analysis: An Essay on the Organization of Experience*, Harmondsworth: Penguin Books.

Goodman, A. (2020) 'Stay home, stay safe, be kind: what New Zealand can teach the world about eliminating COVID-19', *democracynow*, 26 May, Available from: www.democracynow.org/2020/5/26/new_zealand_ coronavirus_response_jacinda_ardern [Accessed 15 December 2020].

Government of Canada (2020) 'Coronavirus disease (COVID-19): prevention and risks', Available from: www.canada.ca/en/public-health/services/disea ses/2019-novel-coronavirus-infection/prevention- risks.html [Accessed 13 May 2020].

Gov.UK (2020a) 'Prime minister's statement on coronavirus (COVID-19): 12 March 2020', Available from: https://www.gov.uk/government/ speeches/pm-statement-on-coronavirus-12-march-2020 [Accessed 21 September 2022].

Gov.UK (2020b) 'Prime minister's statement on coronavirus (COVID-19): 16 March 2020', Available from: https://www.gov.uk/government/speeches/ pm-statement-on-coronavirus-16-march-2020 [Accessed 21 September 2022].

Gov.UK (2020c) 'New campaign to prevent spread of coronavirus indoors this winter: Press Release', Department of Health and Social Care, 9 September, Available from: https://www.gov.uk/government/news/new- campaign-to-prevent-spread-of-coronavirus-indoors-this-winter [Accessed 5 December 2022].

Gov.UK (2021a) 'UK summary: the official UK government website for data and insights on coronavirus (COVID-19), 25 August 2021', Available from: https://coronavirus.data.gov.uk [Accessed 25 August 2021].

Gov.UK (2021b) 'Vaccinations in United Kingdom', Gov.UK, 3 October, Available from: https://coronavirus.data.gov.uk/details/vaccinations [Accessed 4 October 2021].

Gov.UK (2021c) 'Chief Medical Officer: Professor Chris Whitty', Available from: https://www.gov.uk/government/people/christopher-whitty#previ ous-roles [Accessed 1 November 2021].

Gov.UK (2021d) 'Chief Executive: Dr Jenny Harries', Available from: https://www.gov.uk/government/people/jenny-harries [Accessed 1 November 2021].

Gov.UK (2021e) 'List of membership of SAGE and related sub-groups', updated 18 June, Available from: https://www.gov.uk/government/ publications/scientific-advisory-group-for-emergencies-sage-coronavi rus-covid-19-response-membership/list-of-participants-of-sage-and-rela ted-sub-groups [Accessed 2 November 2021].

Gov.UK (2021f) 'Independent report: JCVI statement on COVID-19 vaccination of children aged 12 to 15 years: 3 September 2021', Available from: https://www.gov.uk/government/publications/jcvi-statement- september-2021-covid-19-vaccination-of-children-aged-12-to-15-years/ jcvi-statement-on-covid-19-vaccination-of-children-aged-12-to-15-years- 3-september-2021 [Accessed 3 November 2021].

Gov.UK (2021g) 'New campaign to "Stop COVID-19 hanging around"', press release, Department of Health and Social Care, 5 November, Available from: https://www.gov.uk/government/news/new-campaign-to-stop-covid-19-hanging-around [Accessed 29 November 2021].

Gov.UK (2021h) 'Prime minister announces Covid-19 inquiry chair', 15 December 2021, Available from: https://www.gov.uk/government/news/prime-minister-announces-covid-19-inquiry-chair [Accessed 31 January 2022].

Gov.UK (2022a) 'Coronavirus (COVID-19) in the UK', 6 April, Available from: https://coronavirus.data.gov.uk [Accessed 7 April 2022, note these data were valid on this date but the site was updated daily].

Gov.UK (2022b) 'COVID-19 confirmed deaths in England (to 31 January 2022): report', updated 3 May, Available from: https://www.gov.uk/government/publications/covid-19-reported-sars-cov-2-deaths-in-england/covid-19-confirmed-deaths-in-england-to-31-january-2022-report [Accessed 27 June 2022].

Government of Japan (2020) 'Expert Meeting on the Novel Coronavirus Disease Control "Views on the Novel Coronavirus Disease Control"', 9 March, Available from: https://www.mhlw.go.jp/content/10900000/000608425.pdf [Accessed 5 August 2021].

Grattan, M. (2020) 'Scott Morrison indicates 'eliminating' COVID-19 would come at too high a cost', *The Conversation*, 7 April, Available from: https://theconversation.com/scott-morrison-indicates-eliminating-covid-19-would-come-at-too-high-a-cost-135857 [Accessed 19 August 2021].

Great Barrington Declaration (2020) 'Great Barrington Declaration', Available from: https://gbdeclaration.org [Accessed 13 September 2021].

Green, J. (1999) 'From accidents to risk: public health and preventable injury', *Health, Risk & Society*, 1(1): 25–39.

Greenhalgh, T., Ozbilgin, M. and Contandriopoulos, D. (2021) 'Orthodoxy, *illusio*, and playing the scientific game: a Bourdieusian analysis of infection control science in the COVID-19 pandemic', *Wellcome Open Research*, 6(126), Available from: https://wellcomeopenresearch.org/articles/6-126/v3 [Accessed 3 January 2022].

Griglio, E. (2020) 'Parliamentary oversight under the Covid-19 emergency: striving against executive dominance', *The Theory and Practice of Legislation*, 8(1–2): 49–70, Available from: https://doi.org/10.1080/20508840.2020.1789935 [Accessed 3 January 2022].

The Guardian (2021) 'Lost to the virus', *The Guardian*, Available from: https://www.theguardian.com/society/series/lost-to-the-virus [Accessed 17 December 2021].

Hackel, J. (2020) 'Fauci shuns Trump's politicization of COVID-19 science to focus on "public health message"', *The World*, 13 October, Available from: https://www.pri.org/stories/2020-10-13/fauci-shuns-trumps-politicization-covid-19-science-focus-public-health-message [Accessed 28 October 2021].

Haddon, C. (2021) 'COBR (COBRA)', Institute for Government, 30 March 2021, Available from: https://www.instituteforgovernment.org. uk/explainers/cobr-cobra [Accessed 3 November 2020].

Haider, N. et al (2020) 'Lockdown measures in response to COVID-19 in nine sub-Saharan African countries', *BMJ Global Health*, 5:e003319, Available from: https://gh.bmj.com/content/bmjgh/5/10/e003319.full. pdf [Accessed 17 June 2022].

Hancock, M. (2020a) Twitter, 24 January, Available from: https://twitter. com/matthancock/status/1220722805551124483?lang=en [Accessed 5 December 2022].

Hancock, M. (2020b) 'Health and Social Care Secretary's statement on coronavirus (COVID-19): 15 April 2020', Available from: www.gov.uk/gov ernment/speeches/health-and-social-care-secretarys-statement-on-coro navirus-covid-19-15-april-2020 [Accessed 15 December 2020].

Hancock, M. (2021a) 'How we got here: lessons from the UK vaccine rollout: speech by Secretary of State for Health and Social Care Matt Hancock at the Jenner Institute Laboratories, University of Oxford, 2 June 2021', Available from: https://www.gov.uk/government/speeches/ how-we-got-here-lessons-from-the-uk-vaccine-rollout [Accessed 14 August 2021].

Hancock, M. (2021b) 'Secretary of State for Health, Matt Hancock, on ME/ CFS & COVID vaccine priority', 19 February, Available from: https:// meassociation.org.uk/2021/02/matt-hancock-on-me-cfs-covid-vaccine- priority/ [Accessed 18 August 2022].

Harlan, C. and Pitrelli, S. (2020) 'As coronavirus cases grow, hospitals in northern Italy are running out of beds', *Washington Post*, 12 March, Available from: https://www.washingtonpost.com/world/europe/italy- coronavirus-patients-lombardy-hospitals/2020/03/12/36041dc6-63ce- 11ea-8a8e-5c5336b32760_story.html [Accessed 8 March 2021].

Harries, T. (2008) 'Feeling secure or being secure? Why it can seem better not to protect yourself against a natural hazard', *Health, Risk & Society*, 10(5): 479–90.

Hart, R. (2021) 'Fauci says military who refuse Covid-19 vaccine are 'part of the problem' after high rate of service members refuse jab', *Forbes*, 5 March, Available from: https://www.forbes.com/sites/roberthart/2021/ 03/05/fauci-says-military-who-refuse-covid-19-vaccine-are-part-of-the- problem-after-high-rate-of-service-members-refuse-jab/?sh=4de0e145b b4a [Accessed 30 September 2021].

Health and Social Care Committee (2020) 'Oral evidence: coronavirus – NHS preparedness', HC 36, 17 March, Available from: https://committ ees.parliament.uk/oralevidence/208/pdf/ [Accessed 8 March 2021].

Hersche, B., Kern, W., Stuber-Berries, N., Rohrer, R., Trkola, A. and Weber, K. (2020) 'Bericht der Unabhängigen Expertenkommission: Management Covid-19-Pandemie Tirol', 12 October, Available from: www.tirol.gv.at/presse/webinar-land-tirol/expertenkommission/ [Accessed 15 December 2020].

Heyman, B., Shaw, B., Alaszewski, A. and Titterton, M. (2010) *Risk, Safety and Clinical Practice: Health Care through the Lens of Risk*, Oxford: Oxford University Press.

Hindhede, A.L. (2014) 'Prediabetic categorisation: the making of a new person', *Health, Risk & Society*, 16 (7–8): 600–14.

HM Government (2022) *COVID-19 Response: Living with COVID-19*, Available from: https://assets.publishing.service.gov.uk/government/uploads/system/uploads/attachment_data/file/1056229/COVID-19_Response_-_Living_with_COVID-19.pdf [Accessed 8 April 2022].

HM Treasury (2005) *Managing Risks to the Public: Appraisal Guidance*, London, HMSO, Available from: https://assets.publishing.service.gov.uk/government/uploads/system/uploads/attachment_data/file/191518/Managing_risks_to_the_public_appraisal_guidance.pdf [Accessed 11 October 2021].

Holmes, C.A. and Warelow, P. (1999) 'Implementing psychiatry as risk management: DSM-IV as a postmodern taxonomy', *Health, Risk & Society*, 1(2): 167–78.

Honigsbaum, M. (2020) *The Pandemic Century: A History of Global Contagion from the Spanish Flu to Covid-19* (revised ed.), London: Penguin Random House.

Horlick-Jones, T. (2005) 'On "risk work": professional discourse, accountability, and everyday action'. *Health, Risk & Society*, 7(3): 293–307.

Horton, R. (2020) *The COVID-19 Catastrophe: What's Gone Wrong and How to Stop it Happening Again*, Cambridge: Polity Press.

House Committee on Transportation and Infrastructure (2020) *The Design, Development and Certification of the Boeing 737 Max*, Available from: https://transportation.house.gov/imo/media/doc/2020.09.15%20FINAL%20737%20MAX%20Report%20 for%20Public%20Release.pdf [Accessed 15 December 2020].

House of Commons, Health and Social Care Committee and Science and Technology Committee (2021a) 'Oral evidence: coronavirus: lessons learnt', HC 95, Wednesday 26 May, London: House of Commons, Available from: https://committees.parliament.uk/oralevidence/2249/html/ [Accessed 1 February 2022].

House of Commons, Health and Social Care Committee and Science and Technology Committee (2021b) *Coronavirus: Lessons Learned to Date*, London: House of Commons, Available from: https://publications.parliament.uk/pa/cm5802/cmselect/cmsctech/92/9203.htm [Accessed 1 February 2022].

House of Commons, Committee on Science and Technology (2021) 'The UK response to covid-19: use of scientific evidence', HC 136, 8 January, Available from: https://publications.parliament.uk/pa/cm5801/cmselect/cmsctech/136/136.pdf [Accessed 3 November 2021].

House of Commons, Public Accounts Committee (2020) 'Readying the NHS and social care for the COVID-19 peak', HC 405, Available from: https://committees.parliament.uk/publications/2179/documents/20139/default/ [Accessed 3 November 2021].

Hung, Y.W. (2020) 'Creative public-private collaborations in Taiwan and South Korea bolster the fight against coronavirus', *Stanford Social Innovation Review*, Available from: https://ssir.org/articles/entry/creative_public_private_collaborations_in_taiwan_and_south_korea_bolster_the_fight_against_coronavirus [Accessed 15 December 2020].

IC (2021) 'Unclassified summary of assessment on COVID-19 origins', Available from: https://www.dni.gov/files/ODNI/documents/assessments/Unclassified-Summary-of-Assessment-on-COVID-19-Origins.pdf [Accessed 5 December 2022].

Imai, N., Dorigatti, I., Cori, A., Riley, S. and Ferguson, N.M. (2020) *Report 1: Estimating the Potential Total Number of Novel Coronavirus Cases in Wuhan City, China*, Imperial College London COVID-19 Response Team, Available from: www.imperial.ac.uk/media/imperial-college/medicine/mrc-gida/2020-01-17-COVID19-Report-1.pdf [Accessed 15 December 2020].

Independent Panel [for Pandemic Preparedness and Response] (2021) *COVID-19: Making it the Last Pandemic*, Available from: https://theindependentpanel.org/wp-content/uploads/2021/05/COVID-19-Make-it-the-Last-Pandemic_final.pdf [Accessed 19 July 2021].

Insight (2020) 'A weeping nurse said, "They are all going to die – no one is doing anything about it"', *Sunday Times*, 25 October, pp 7–11.

Ittefaq, M., Hussain, S.A. and Fatima, M. (2020) 'COVID-19 and social-politics of medical disinformation in social media in Pakistan', *Media Asia*, 47(1–2): 75–80.

Jabs (2011) 'Welcome to the support group for vaccine damaged children', Available from: www.jabs.org.uk [Accessed 18 January 2011].

Jabs (2020) 'Graham Hutchinson, ex-Senior Chief Biomedical Scientist, Public Health UK – 5th November 2020', Available from: http://www.jabs.org.uk [Accessed 1 December 2020].

Jabs (2022) 'Home news', Available from: http://www.jabs.org.uk [Accessed 5 September 2022].

Jackson, B. and Pederson, A.B. (2020) 'Facing both Covid-19 and racism, Black women are carrying a particularly heavy burden', *Washington Post*, 4 September, Available from: www.washington-post.com/opinions/2020/09/04/facing-both-covid-19-racism- black-women-are-carrying-particularly-heavy-burden/ [Accessed 15 December 2020].

Japanese Times (2020) 'Japan confirms first case of coronavirus that has infected dozens in China', *Japanese Times*, 16 January, Available from: www.japantimes.co.jp/news/2020/01/16/national/science-health/japan-first-coronavirus-case/ [Accessed 15 December 2020].

JCVI (2020a) 'Advice on priority groups for COVID-19 vaccination', 2 December, Available from: https://assets.publishing.service.gov.uk/gov ernment/uploads/system/uploads/attachment_data/file/940936/Priority_groups_for_coronavirus__COVID-19__vaccination_-_advice_from_the_JCVI__2_December_2020.pdf [Accessed 15 December 2020].

JCVI (2020b) 'Joint committee on vaccination and immunisation', Available from: www.gov.uk/government/groups/joint-committee-on-vaccination-and-immunisation [Accessed 15 December 2020].

Jennings, W., Vagardsson, V., Stoker, G et al (2020) 'Political trust and the COVID-19 crisis: pushing populism to the backburner', Democracy 2025, Available from: https://www.ipsos.com/sites/default/files/ct/news/documents/2020-08/covid_and_trust.pdf [Accessed 14 September 2022].

Jerusalem Post Staff (2020) 'Pakistani cleric: Jews are responsible for creation of coronavirus', *Jerusalem Post*, 8 May 2020, Available from: https://www.jpost.com/international/pakistani-cleric-jews-are-responsible-for-creat ion-of-coronavirus-627333 [Accessed 2 September 2022].

Jetten, J., Reicher, S.D., Haslam, S.A. and Cruwys, T. (2020) *Together Apart: The Psychology of Covid-19*, London and Thousand Oaks, CA: Sage.

Johns Hopkins University of Medicine (2021) 'Mortality analyses', Available from: https://coronavirus.jhu.edu/data/mortality [Accessed 27 September 2021].

Johns Hopkins University of Medicine (2022) 'Mortality analyses', Available from: https://coronavirus.jhu.edu/data/mortality [Accessed 28 February 2022].

Johnson, B. (2020a) 'Prime minister's statement on coronavirus (COVID-19): 12 October 2020', Available from: https://www.gov.uk/government/speeches/prime-ministers-statement-on-coronavirus-covid-19-12-octo ber-2020 [Accessed 20 August 2021].

Johnson, B. (2020c) 'Prime minister's statement on coronavirus (COVID-19): 31 October 2020', Available from: https://www.gov.uk/government/speeches/prime-ministers-statement-on-coronavirus-covid-19-31-octo ber-2020 [Accessed 20 August 2021].

Johnson, B. (2020d) 'Prime minister's statement on coronavirus (COVID-19): 19 December 2020', Available from: https://www.gov.uk/governm ent/speeches/prime-ministers-statement-on-coronavirus-covid-19-19-december-2020 [Accessed 23 August 2021].

Johnson, B. (2021a) 'Prime minister sets out roadmap to cautiously ease lockdown restrictions', 22 February 2021, Available from: https://www.gov.uk/government/news/prime-minister-sets-out-roadmap-to-cautiou sly-ease-lockdown-restrictions [Accessed 23 August 2021].

Johnson, B. (2021b) 'Press release: vaccination programme accelerated as Step 4 is paused', 14 June 2021, Available from: https://www.gov.uk/gov ernment/news/vaccination-programme-accelerated-as-step-4-is-paused [Accessed 23 August 2021].

Johnson, B. (2021c) 'PM statement at coronavirus press conference: 12 July 2021', Available from: https://www.gov.uk/government/speeches/ pm-statement-at-coronavirus-press-conference-12-july-2021 [Accessed 23 August 2021].

Johnson, B. (2021d) 'PM statement at coronavirus press conference: 19 July 2021', Available from: https://www.gov.uk/government/speeches/ pm-statement-at-coronavirus-press-conference-19-july-2021 [Accessed 24 August 2021].

Johnson, B. (2021e) 'Prime minister's address to the nation', 12 December 2021, Available from: https://www.gov.uk/government/speeches/prime-ministers-address-to-the-nation-on-booster-jabs-12-december-2021 [Accessed 17 April 2022].

Johnson, V. (2020b) 'When it comes to coronavirus, Ardern is winning on the world stage', *stuff*, 27 March, Available from: www.stuff.co.nz/national/ politics/opinion/120590435/in-the-survivor-jungle-ardern-is-winning-the-communications-contest [Accessed 15 December 2020].

Joint Inquiry [the House Permanent Select Committee on Intelligence and the Senate Select Committee on Intelligence] (2002) Report of the Joint Inquiry into the Terrorist Attacks of September 11, 2001, Available from: https://www.intelligence.senate.gov/sites/default/files/documents/ CRPT-107srpt351-5.pdf [Accessed 4 May 2022].

Joint Working Party [of Members of the Standing Committee on Vaccination, the German Ethics Council and the National Academy of Sciences Leopoldina] (2020) 'How should access to a COVID-19 vaccine be regulated?', 9 November, Available from: https://www.ethikrat.org/ fileadmin/Publikationen/Ad-hoc-Empfehlungen/englisch/joint-posit ion-paper-stiko-der-leopoldina-vaccine-prioritisation.pdf [Accessed 20 September 2020].

Jordan, D. (2019) 'The deadliest flu: the complete story of the discovery and reconstruction of the 1918 pandemic virus', Available from: https:// www.cdc.gov/flu/pandemic-resources/reconstruction-1918-virus.html [Accessed 2 December 2022].

Jurich, E.K. (2021) '"Do you think this is normal?": risk, temporality, and the management of children's food allergies through online support groups', *Health, Risk and Society*, 23(3–4): 128–42.

Kahne, J. and Bowyer, B. (2018) 'The political significance of social media activity and social networks', *Political Communication*, 35(3): 470–93.

Kaiser, C. (2022) 'The Storm is Upon Us review: indispensable QAnon history', updated, *The Guardian*, 21 August, Available from: https://www.theguardian.com/books/2022/aug/21/the-storm-is-upon-us-review-qanon-history-updated-trump-january-6 [Accessed 4 September 2022].

Kakimoto, K., Kamiya, H., Yamagishi, T., Matsui, T., Suzuki, M. and Wakita, T. (2020) 'Initial investigation of transmission of COVID-19 among crew members during quarantine of a cruise ship – Yokohama, Japan, February 2020', *Morbidity and Mortality Weekly Reports* (CDC), 69(11): 312–13, Available from: https://pubmed.ncbi.nlm.nih.gov/32191689/ [Accessed 6 April 2022].

Kale, S. (2021) 'Lost to the virus: Samantha Willis was a beloved young pregnant mother. Did bad vaccine advice cost her her life?' *The Guardian*, 23 November, Available from: https://www.theguardian.com/society/2021/nov/23/samantha-willis-was-a-beloved-young-pregnant-mother-did-bad-vaccine-advice-cost-her-her-life [Accessed 10 January 2022].

Kermani, S. (2020) 'Coronavirus: Whitty and Vallance faced "herd immunity" backlash, emails show', BBC, 23 September, Available from: www.bbc.co.uk/news/uk-politics-54252272 [Accessed 15 December 2020].

Kewell, B.J. (2006) 'Language games and tragedy: the Bristol Royal Infirmary disaster revisited', *Health, Risk & Society*, 8(4): 359–77.

Kiisel, M. and Vihalemm, T. (2014) 'Why the transformation of the risk message is a healthy sign: a model of the reception of warning messages', *Health, Risk & Society*, 16(3): 277–94.

Kilbourne, E.D. (2006) 'Influenza pandemics of the 20th century', *Emerging Infectious Diseases*, 12(1): 9–14, Available from: https://www.ncbi.nlm.nih.gov/pmc/articles/PMC3291411/ [Accessed 6 August 2021].

Kim, J.H. and Scialli, A.R. (2011) 'Thalidomide: the tragedy of birth defects and the effective treatment of disease', *Toxicological Science*, 122(1): 1–6.

Kim, J.-H., An, J. A.-R., Oh, S.J.J., Oh, J. and Lee, J.-K.(2021) 'Emerging COVID-19 success story: South Korea learned the lessons of MERS', *Our World in Data*, 5 March, Available from: https://ourworldindata.org/covid-exemplar-south-korea [Accessed 6 June 2022].

Knapton, S. (2020) '"Rash" northern lockdown based on inaccurate data, says expert', *Daily Telegraph*, 3 August, Available from: www.telegraph.co.uk/news/2020/08/02/lockdown-north-england-rash-decision-not-backed-data-oxford/ [Accessed 15 December 2020].

Knight, M. et al (2020) 'Characteristics and outcomes of pregnant women admitted to hospital with confirmed SARS-CoV-2 infection in UK: national population based cohort study', *BMJ*, 369, Available from: www.bmj.com/content/369/bmj.m2107 [Accessed 6 August 2020].

Kontopantelis, E., Mamas, M.A., Deanfield, J., Asaria, M. and Doran, T.(2021) 'Excess mortality in England and Wales during the first wave of the COVID-19 pandemic', *Epidemiology and Community, Health*, 75: 213–23, Available from: https://jech.bmj.com/content/75/3/213 [Accessed 19 August 2021].

Kriesi, H. (2014) 'The populist challenge', *West European Politics*, 37(2): 361–78.

Learn The Risk (n.d.) 'Learn The risk.Org: Knowledge • Action • Health', Available from: https://learntherisk.org [Accessed 15 December 2020].

Lebela, C., MacKinnin, A., Bagshawe, M., Tomfohr-Madsen, L. and Giesbrecht, G. (2020) 'Elevated depression and anxiety symptoms among pregnant individuals during the COVID-19 pandemic', *Journal of Affective Disorders*, 277: 5–13.

Lewis, G. (2000) *A Failure of Treatment*, Oxford: Oxford University Press.

Lewis, D. (2020) 'Why many countries failed at COVID contact-tracing – but some got it right', *Nature*, 17 December, 588: 384–7, Available from: https://media.nature.com/original/magazine-assets/d41 586-020-03518-4/d41586-020-03518-4.pdf [Accessed 5 August 2020].

Lewison, G. (2008) 'The reporting of the risks from severe acute respiratory syndrome (SARS) in the news media, 2003–2004', *Health, Risk and Society*, 10(3): 241–2.

Lindsay, B. (2020) 'Controversy over airborne transmission of COVID-19 "a tempest in a teapot," Dr. Bonnie Henry says', CBC News, 7 July, Available from: https://www.cbc.ca/news/canada/controversy-over-airborne-trans mission-of-covid-19-a-tempest-in-a-teapot-dr-bonnie-henry-says-1.5639 958 [Accessed 30 November 2020].

Litvinova, D. (2020) 'Putin orders "large-scale" COVID-19 vaccination in Russia', Associated Press, 2 December, Available from: www. sfgate. com/news/article/Putin-orders-large-scale-vaccination-of-15769550.php [Accessed 15 December 2020].

Llupià, A., Rodríguez-Giralt, I., Fité, A,. Álamo, L., de la Torre, L., Redondo, A., Callau, M. and Guinovart, C. (2020) 'What is a zero-COVID strategy and how can it help us minimise the impact of the pandemic', Institute for Global Health, Barcelona, 26, 27 November, Available from: https://www.isglobal.org/en_GB/-/-que-es-una-estrate gia-de-covid-cero-y-como-puede-ayudarnos-a-minimizar-el-impacto-de-la-pandemia- [Accessed 4 August 2021].

Luhmann, N. (1993) *Risk: A Sociological Theory*, Berlin: de Gruyter.

Lupton, D. (1999) *Risk and Sociocultural Theory: New Directions and Perspectives*, Cambridge: Cambridge University Press.

Mackintosh, T. (2020) 'Coronavirus: the London hospital hit by a "tidal wave" of patients', BBC News, 2 June, Available from: https://www.bbc. co.uk/news/uk-england-london-52812457 [Accessed 9 March 2021].

Mairal, G. (2011) 'The history and the narrative of risk in the media', *Health, Risk & Society*, 13(1): 65–79.

Mance, H. (2016) 'Britain has had enough of experts, says Gove', *Financial Times*, 3 June, Available from: www.ft.com/con-tent/3be49734-29cb-11e6-83e4-abc22d5d108c [Accessed 15 December 2020].

Mao, F. (2022) 'China abandons key parts of zero-Covid strategy after protests', BBC News, 7 December, Available from: https://www.bbc.co.uk/news/world-asia-china-63855508 [Accessed 8 December 2022].

Martin, S. (2021) 'Scott Morrison criticises plan to pursue Covid-zero strategy even when vaccination high as "absurd"', *The Guardian*, 16 August, Available from: https://www.theguardian.com/australia-news/2021/aug/16/scott-morrison-criticises-was-absurd-plan-to-pursue-covid-zero-strat egy-even-when-vaccination-high [Accessed 1 April 2022].

Matar, R., Alrahmani, L., Monzer, N. Debiane, L.G., Berban, E., Fares, J. Fitzpatrick, F. and Murad, M.H. (2020) Clinical Presentation and Outcomes of Pregnant Women With Coronavirus Disease 2019: A Systematic Review and Meta-analysis, *Clinical Infectious Diseases*, 23 June, ciaa828, Available from: https://www.ncbi.nlm.nih.gov/pmc/articles/PMC7337 697/ [Accessed 15 September 2020].

Maxmen, A. and Mallapaty, S. (2021) 'The COVID lab-leak hypothesis: what scientists do and don't know', *Nature, New Explainer*, 8 June, Available from: https://www.nature.com/articles/d41586-021-01529-3 [10 July 2021].

Mazza, E. (2020) 'Trump's bonkers coronavirus "herd mentality" claim lights up Twitter', *HuffPost US*, 16 September, Available from: www.huf fingtonpost.co.uk/entry/donald-trump-herd-mentality_n_5f618e1ac5b6e 27db134a42b?ri18n=true [Accessed 15 December 2020].

McClure, T. (2021) 'Ardern's Covid lockdown finds favour as New Zealand watches Sydney's Delta disaster', *The Guardian*, 18 August 2021, Available from: https://www.theguardian.com/world/2021/aug/18/arderns-covid-lockdown-finds-favour-as-new-zealand-watches-sydneys-delta-disaster [Accessed 18 August 2021].

McGrath, B. (2020) 'Japanese government facing growing criticism over Covid-19 outbreak', *World Socialist Website*, Available from: www.wsws.org/en/articles/2020/03/03/japa-m03.html [Accessed 15 December 2020].

McMullen, J. (2020) 'Covid-19: Five days that shaped the outbreak', BBC News, 26 January, Available from: https://www.bbc.co.uk/news/world-55756452 [Accessed 1 December 2020].

Mihelj, S., Kondor, K. and Štětka, V. (2022) 'Establishing trust in experts during a crisis: expert trustworthiness and media use during the COVID-19 pandemic', *Science Communication*, 44(3): 292–319.

Mitchell, H. (2017) 'Sierra Leone: teenage girls are dying from unsafe abortions and risky pregnancies', *The Guardian,* 20 July, available from: https://www.theguardian.com/global-development-profession als-network/2017/jul/20/teen-pregnancy-sierra-leone-involve-men [Accessed 1 June 2020].

Mohan, G. (2014) 'With Ebola cases, CDC zeros in on lapses in protocol, protective gear', *Los Angeles Times*, 15 October, Available from: https://www.latimes.com/nation/la-na-ebola-protocols-20141015-story.html [Accessed 11 March 2021].

Mohdin, A. (2020) '"He was full of hope": stories behind five of the 3,173 UK Covid deaths this summer', *The Guardian*, 13 October, Available from: www.theguardian.com/world/2020/oct/13/he-was-full-of-hope-five-uk-covid-deaths-summer-stories [Accessed 3 February 2021].

Mogelson, L. (2022) '"American rebellion": the lockdown protests that paved the way for the Capitol riots', *The Observer*, 28 August, Available from: https://www.theguardian.com/us-news/2022/aug/28/luke-mogelson-the-storm-is-here-capitol-attack-michigan-book [Accessed 4 September 2022].

Möllering, G. (2001) 'The nature of trust: from Georg Simmel to a theory of expectation, interpretation and suspension', *Sociology*, 35(2): 403–20.

Morelle, R. (2020) 'Covid test-and-trace: is backwards contact tracing the way forward?' BBC News, 6 December, Available from: https://www.bbc.co.uk/news/health-54648734 [Accessed 5 August 2021].

Morgan, P. (2021) Twitter, 19 July, Available from: https://twitter.com/piersmorgan/status/1417098654435921922?lang=en [Accessed 15 September 2021].

Morowska, L. and Milton, D.K. (2020) 'It is time to address airborne transmission of Coronavirus Disease 2019 (COVID-19)', *Clinical Infectious Diseases*, 6 July, 71(9): 2311–13, Available from: https://academic.oup.com/cid/article/71/9/2311/5867798 [Accessed 1 July 2022].

Mulkay, M.J. (1979) *Science and the Sociology of Knowledge*, London: G. Allen & Unwin.

NERVTAG (2015) '1st annual report December 2014–December 2015', Available from: https://app.box.com/s/qdlzn521h06891utpzqlfo9svy4wn u0d/file/73089104785 [Accessed 2 November 2021].

New York Times (2020) 'Full transcript: Trump's 2020 State of the Union address, 5 February 2020', Available from: https://www.nytimes.com/2020/02/05/us/politics/state-of-union-transcript.html [Accessed 16 February 2022].

New York Times (2021) 'Tracking coronavirus vaccinations around the world', Available from: https://www.nytimes.com/interactive/2021/world/covid-vaccinations-tracker.html [Accessed 16 August 2021].

New Zealand Cabinet Office (2020) 'Update on novel coronavirus: Infectious and Notifiable Diseases Order 2020', Cabinet Office, Minute of Decision, Available from: https://covid19.govt.nz/assets/resources/proactive-rele ase/Update-on-Novel-Coronavirus- Infectious-and-Notifiable-Diseases- Order-2020-Minute-28-01- 20.pdf [Accessed 15 December 2020].

New Zealand Government (2020) 'Alert system overview: New Zealand's 4-level alert system lists the measures to be taken against COVID-19 at each level', Available from: https://covid19.govt.nz/alert-system/alert-sys tem-overview/#alert-level-1-—-prepare [Accessed 15 December 2020].

New Zealand Ministry of Health (2021) 'COVID-19 (novel coronavirus)', Available from: https://www.health.govt.nz/our-work/diseases-and-con ditions/covid-19-novel-coronavirus [Accessed 17 August 2021].

NHS (2021) 'Quarterly attendances & emergency admission monthly statistics, NHS and independent sector organisations in England', 14 January, Available from: https://www.england.nhs.uk/statistics/statisti cal-work-areas/ae-waiting-times-and-activity/ [Accessed 8 March 2021].

NICE (2020) Twitter, 13 April, Available from: https://twitter.com/niceco mms/status/1249650194804850689 [Accessed 20 April 2022].

Nigeria Centre for Disease Control and Prevention (2022) Home page, Available from: https://ncdc.gov.ng [Accessed 4 December 2022].

NIHR (2022) 'National Institute for Health and Care Research', Available from: https://www.nihr.ac.uk [Accessed 9 August 2022].

NPHIL (2021) 'National Public Health Institute Liberia', Available from: https://www.nphil.gov.lr/index.php/about-us/ [Accessed 12 October 2021].

New Zealand Herald (2020) 'Covid 19 coronavirus: New Zealanders' trust in Government's pandemic management falls', *New Zealand Herald*, 8 August 2020, Available from: www.nzherald.co.nz/nz/covid-19-coronavirus-new- zealanders-trust-in-governments-pandemic-management-falls/ [Accessed 15 December 2020].

Novel Coronavirus Pneumonia Emergency Response Epidemiology Team (2020) 'The epidemiological characteristics of an outbreak of 2019 novel coronavirus diseases (COVID-19) — China, 2020', *China CDC Weekly*, 2(8): 113–22, Available from: https://weekly.chinacdc.cn/en/article/doi/ 10.46234/ccdcw2020.032 [Accessed 4 April 2022].

Obama, B. (2020) 'Barack Obama talks to David Olusoga', 19 November, *BBC Sounds*, Available from: www.bbc.co.uk/sounds/series/m000q57g [Accessed 15 December 2020].

Odour, M. (2021) 'Tanzania still in denial about Covid-19 existence despite surge in cases', AfricaNews, 18 February, Available from: https://www.afr icanews.com/2021/02/18/tanzania-still-in-denial-about-covid-19-exista nce-despite-surge-in-cases// [Accessed 14 October 2021].

O'Grady, S. (2022) 'Why Boris Johnson and the government can't just 'move on' from Partygate', *The Independent*, 30 May, Available from: https://www.independent.co.uk/independentpremium/politics-explained/boris-johnson-mps-partygate-b2090480.html [Accessed 23 June 2022].

OECD (2021) 'Enhancing public trust in COVID-19 vaccination: the role of governments', OECD, 10 May, Available from: https://www.oecd.org/coronavirus/policy-responses/enhancing-public-trust-in-covid-19-vaccination-the-role-of-governments-eae0ec5a/ [Accessed 4 October 2021].

ONS (2019) 'Families and households in the UK: 2019', ONS, Available from: https://www.ons.gov.uk/peoplepopulationandcommunity/birthsdeathsandmarriages/families/bulletins/familiesandhouseholds/2019#toc [Accessed 8 March 2021].

ONS (2021a) 'Coronavirus and vaccine hesitancy, Great Britain: 9 August 2021', ONS, Available from: https://www.ons.gov.uk/peoplepopulationandcommunity/healthandsocialcare/healthandwellbeing/bulletins/coronavirusandvaccinehesitancygreatbritain/9august2021 [Accessed 4 October 2021].

ONS (2021b) 'Coronavirus and vaccination rates in people aged 50 years and over by socio-demographic characteristic, England: 8 December 2020 to 12 April 2021', ONS, Available from: https://www.ons.gov.uk/peoplepopulationandcommunity/healthandsocialcare/healthinequalities/bulletins/coronavirusandvaccinationratesinpeopleaged70yearsandoverbysociodemographiccharacteristicengland/8december2020to12april2021 [Accessed 4 October 2021].

O'Toole, F. (2018) *Heroic Failure: Brexit and the Politics of Pain*, London: Head of Zeus.

Parsley, D. (2021) 'Boris Johnson "privately accepts" up to 50,000 annual Covid deaths as an acceptable level', *The Independent*, 27 August, Available from: https://inews.co.uk/news/boris-johnson-privately-accepts-up-to-50000-annual-covid-deaths-as-an-acceptable-level-1170069 [Accessed 30 August 2021].

Parveen, N. (2020a) '"What is happening is not normal. We 100% need answers. This is not adding up"', *The Guardian*, 22 April, Available from: www.theguardian.com/world/2020/apr/22/what-is-happening-is-not-normal-we-100-need-answers-this-is-not-adding-up [Accessed 15 December 2020].

Parveen, N. (2020b) 'Dominic Cummings row: senior health official says lockdown rules "apply to all"', *The Guardian*, 30 May, Available from: https://www.theguardian.com/world/2020/may/30/dominic-cummings-jonathan-van-tam-lockdown-rules-apply-to-all [Accessed 2 November 2021].

Patil, A. (2021) '"Captain Tom," the 100-year-old who raised millions for Britain's health system, gets a hero's goodbye at his funeral', *New York Times*, 27 February, Available from: https://www.nytimes.com/2021/02/27/world/captain-tom-moore-funeral.html [Accessed 18 December 2021].

Paton, A. (2020) 'Vaccine should go to those most in need', *The Independent*, 11 November, p. 9.

Penna, D. (2020) 'Captain Tom Moore knighted by the Queen and jokes: "If I kneel down I'll never get up again"', 18 July, *The Telegraph*, Available from: www.telegraph.co.uk/news/2020/07/17/captain-tom-moore-kni ghthood-sir-knighted-queen-ceremony/ [Accessed 15 December 2020].

Phillips, T. (2021) 'Brazil begins parliamentary inquiry into Bolsonaro's Covid response', *The Guardian*, 27 April, Available from: https://www. theguardian.com/world/2021/apr/27/brazil-begins-parliamentary-inqu iry-into-bolsonaros-covid-response [Accessed 29 January 2022].

Philo, G. (ed.) (1996) *Media and Mental Distress*, Harlow: Addison Wesley Longman.

Pietras, E. and Sims, P. (2020) 'Walk of frame: WW2 veteran Tom Moore, 99, raises £7 million for the NHS as he walks 100 laps of his garden', *The Sun*, 15 April, Available from: www.thesun.co.uk/news/11392111/vete ran-99-5-million-nhs/ [Accessed 15 December 2020].

Procopius (1914) *The Persian Wars of Procopius*, Loeb Classical Library, English translation by H.B. Dewing, Available from: https://penelope.uchicago.edu/ Thayer/E/Roman/Texts/Procopius/Wars/2F*.html [Accessed 1 July 2022].

Quigley, K.F. (2005) 'Bug reactions: considering US government and UK government Y2K operations in light of media coverage and public opinion polls', *Health, Risk & Society*, 7(3): 267–91.

Quinn, K. and Papacharissi, Z. (2014). 'The place where our social networks reside: social media and sociality', in M.B. Oliver and A.A. Raney (eds), *Media and Social Life*, New York: Routledge, pp 159–207.

Research America (2018) 'U.S. investments in medical and health research and development, 2013–2017', Available from: https://www.researchamer ica.org/sites/default/files/Policy_Advocacy/2013-2017InvestmentRep ortFall2018.pdf [Accessed 13 October 2021].

Reuters (2020) 'In Peru, bodies mount and masks are reused with region's second highest coronavirus cases', NBC News, 22 April, Available from: https://www.nbcnews.com/news/latino/peru-bodies-mount-masks-are-reused-region-s-second-highest-n1189511 [Accessed 17 June 2022].

Reuters (2021) 'Sydney readies for more military support as delta variant continues to sweep Australia's largest city', CNBC, 12 August, Available from: https://www.cnbc.com/2021/08/13/sydney-readies-for-more-milit ary-support-as-delta-variant-city.html [Accessed 18 August 2021].

Rev (2020a) 'Boris Johnson coronavirus speech transcript: UK PM tells UK to avoid non-essential travel and contact', 17 March, Available from: www. rev.com/blog/transcripts/boris-johnson-coronavirus-speech-transcr ipt-uk-pm-tells-uk-to-avoid-non-essential-travel-contact [Accessed 15 December 2020].

Rev (2020b) 'President Donald Trump and the White House coronavirus task force', 6 April, Available from: https://www.rev.com/transcript-edi tor/shared/4PMxa4rsU1gPWQhG7QH3Ij7EkOsI0TrkYBmSEkJ9bylc Hf48m9NyFcJKz5OMxIxw8D5UKfX5vufJVgVZIVYjI2jUFmM?loadF rom=PastedDeeplink&ts=3701.12 [Accessed 17 March 2021].

Rev (2021) 'Boris Johnson COVID-19 lockdown press conference transcript', 5 January, Available from: www.rev.com/blog/transcripts/ boris-johnson-covid-19-lockdown-press-conference-transcript-january-5 [Accessed 15 December 2021].

Riedel, S. (2005) 'Edward Jenner and the history of smallpox and vaccination', Baylor University Medical Center Proceedings, 18(1): 21–5, Available from: https://www.tandfonline.com/doi/pdf/10.1080/08998 280.2005.11928028 [Accessed 13 January 2022].

Rohrer, R. (2020) 'Report of the Independent Commission of Experts on the management of the COVID-19 pandemic in Tyrol', 12 October, Available from: www.tirol.gv.at/fileadmin/presse/downloads/Presse/Press emappe_englisch.pdf [Accessed 3 February 2021].

Roope, L., Clarke, P. and Duch, R. (2020) 'How should countries roll out Covid-19 vaccine? France and the UK have two different ideas', *The Conversation, Scroll.in*, 18 November, Available from: https://scroll.in/arti cle/978755/how-should-countries-roll-out-covid-19-vaccine-france-and-the-uk-have-two-different-ideas [Accessed 15 December 2020].

Rossen, L.M., Branum, A.M., Ahmad, F.B., Sutton, P. and Anderson, R.N (2020) 'Excess deaths associated with COVID-19, by age and race and ethnicity – United States, January 26–October 3, 2020', *Morbidity and Mortality Weekly Report (MMWR)*, 69(42): 1522–7, Available from: www. cdc.gov/mmwr/volumes/69/wr/mm6942e2.htm?s_cid=mm6942e2_w [Accessed 15 December 2020].

Roth, J.A. (1957) 'Ritual and magic in the control of contagion', *American Sociological Review*, 22(3): 310–14, Available from: https://doi.org/10.2307/ 2088472 [Accessed 1 July 2022].

Roy, E.A. (2020) 'New Zealand health minister demoted after beach visit broke lockdown rules', *The Guardian*, 7 April, Available from: www.theg uardian.com/world/2020/apr/07/new-zealand-health-minister-demoted-after-beach-visit-broke-lockdown-rules [Accessed 15 December 2020].

Rutter, J. (2020) *Remembering the Kindness of Strangers: Division, Unity and Social Connection During and Beyond COVID-19*, London: British Future, Available from: www.britishfuture.org/wp-content/uploads/2020/07/RememberingT heKindnessOfStrangersReport. pdf [Accessed 15 December 2020].

SAGE (2020a) 'Forty-third SAGE meeting on Covid-19, 23rd June', Available from: https://assets.publishing.service.gov.uk/government/uplo ads/system/uploads/attachment_data/file/904665/S0561_Forty-third_SA GE_meeting_on_Covid-19.pdf [Accessed 20 August 2021].

SAGE (2020b) 'Fiftieth SAGE meeting on Covid-19, 6th August 2020', Available from: https://assets.publishing.service.gov.uk/government/uplo ads/system/uploads/attachment_data/file/921205/S0692_Fiftieth_SAGE_ meeting_on_Covid-19.pdf [Accessed 20 August 2021].

SAGE (2020c) 'Sixty-first SAGE meeting on Covid-19, 8th October 2020', Available from: https://assets.publishing.service.gov.uk/government/uplo ads/system/uploads/attachment_data/file/931136/S0800_Sixty-first_SA GE_meeting_on_Covid-19.pdf [Accessed 1 April 2022].

Saleem, A. (2020) 'How denial and conspiracy theories fuel coronavirus crisis in Pakistan', dw.com, Available from: https://www.dw.com/en/how-den ial-and-conspiracy-theories-fuel-coronavirus-crisis-in-pakistan/a-53913 842 [Accessed 1 September 2022].

Sample, I. (2021) 'What are the risks of England unlocking in the Covid third wave?' *The Guardian*, 7 July, Available from: https://www.theguard ian.com/world/2021/jul/07/what-are-the-risks-of-england-unlocking-in-the-covid-third-wave [Accessed 25 August 2021].

Sarris, P. (2021) New approaches to the 'Plague of Justinian', *Past & Present*, gtab024, Available from: https://academic.oup.com/past/advance-article/ doi/10.1093/pastj/gtab024/6427314 [Accessed 1 July 2022].

Sasse, T., Haddon, C. and Nice, A. (2020) *Science Advice in a Crisis*, Institute for Government, Available from: https://www.instituteforgovernment.org. uk/sites/default/files/publications/science-advice-crisis_0.pdf [Accessed 3 November 2021].

Scamell, M. and Alaszewski, A. (2012) 'Fateful moments and the categorisation of risk: midwifery practice and the ever-narrowing window of normality during childbirth', *Health, Risk & Society*, 14(2): 207–21.

Scamell, M. and Stewart, M. (2014) 'Time, risk and midwife practice: the vaginal examination', *Health, Risk & Society*, 16(1): 84–100.

Scientific American (2020) 'From fear to hope', *Scientific American*, 323(4): 12–13, Available from: www.scientificamerican.com/article/sci entific-american-endorses-joe-biden/ [Accessed 15 December 2020].

Scott, D. and Animashuan, C. (2020) 'Covid-19's stunningly unequal death toll in America, in one chart', Vox, 2 October, Available from: www.vox. com/coronavirus-covid19/2020/10/2/21496884/us-covid-19-deaths-by-race-black-white-americans [Accessed 15 December 2020].

Sengupta, K. (2020) 'Coronavirus: inside the UK government's influential behavioural "nudge unit"', *The Independent*, 2 April, Available from: www. independent.co.uk/news/uk/politics/coronavirus-uk-government-nudge-unit-dominic-cummings-herd-immunity-a9444306.html [Accessed 7 April 2020].

Shane, T. (2018) 'The semiotics of authenticity: indexicality in Donald Trump's tweets', *Social Media + Society*, 4(3): 1–18.

Shapiro, E., Brown, E., Lloyd, W. and Miller, A. (2020) 'Faces of some of the lives lost this year in the COVID-19 crisis: those we've lost include Holocaust survivors, war veterans and doctors', ABC News, 26 December, Available from: https://abcnews.go.com/US/faces-coronavirus-pandemic-remembering-died/story?id=69932880 [Accessed 15 December 2020].

Shen, M. (2020) 'Oregon governor declares state of emergency in Portland and says she is "incredibly worried" about violent clashes ahead of Proud Boys rally on Saturday in city plagued by BLM protests', *MailOnline*, 25 September, Available from: www.dailymail.co.uk/news/article-8773871/Oregon-governor-incredibly-worried-violence-Proud-Boys-rally.html [Accessed 15 December 2020].

Shepherd, C. and Riordan, P. (2021) 'China lacks Covid exit strategy as it strives for zero infections', *Financial Times*, 20 July, Available from: https://www.ft.com/content/0f1048e2-62dd-48ae-a80a-6b6b48cc0851 [Accessed 5 August 2021].

Sherman, A. (2020) 'Trump said the Obama admin left him a bare stockpile. Wrong', POLITIFACT, 8 April, Available from: https://www.politifact.com/factchecks/2020/apr/08/donald-trump/trump-said-obama-admin-left-him-bare-stockpile-wro/ [Accessed 8 March 2021].

Shesgreen, D. (2020) 'Senegal's quiet COVID success: test results in 24 hours, temperature checks at every store, no fights over masks', *USA Today*, Available from: https://eu.usatoday.com/story/news/world/2020/09/06/covid-19-why-senegal-outpacing-us-tackling-pandemic/5659696002/ [Accessed 15 December 2020].

Shipman, T. and Wheeler, C. (2020) 'INSIDE NO 10 Coronavirus: ten days that shook Britain – and changed the nation for ever: how Boris Johnson changed his priorities: save lives first, and then salvage the economy', *Sunday Times*. 22 March, Available from: https://www.thetimes.co.uk/article/coronavirus-ten-days-that-shook-britain-and-changed-the-nation-for-ever-spz6sc9vb [Accessed 6 April 2020].

Shimzu, K., Wharton, G., Sakamoto, H. et al, (2020) 'Resurgence of covid-19 in Japan', *BMJ*, 18 August, 370, Available from: https://www.bmj.com/content/370/bmj.m3221 [Accessed 5 August 2021].

Shuster, S. (2020) 'Contagion of fear', *Time*, Available from: https://time.com/wyckoff-hospital-brooklyn-coronavirus/ [Accessed 8 March 2021].

Skandalakis, P.N., Lainas, P.J.E. Skandalakis, J.E. and Mirilas, P. (2006) '"To afford the wounded speedy assistance": Dominique Jean Larrey and Napoleon', *World Journal of Surgery*, 30(8): 1392–9.

Sky News (2020) 'COVID-19: majority of British public do not trust government to manage pandemic – survey', *Sky News*, 6 December, Available from: https://news.sky.com/story/covid-19-majority-of-british-public-do-not-trust-government-to-manage-pandemic-survey-12152793 [Accessed 15 December 2020].

Smyth, C. (2020) 'Coronavirus: No 10 denies Dominic Cummings would have let elderly die', *The Times*, 23 March, Available from: www. thetimes. co.uk/article/no-10-denies-dominic-cummings-would-have-let-elderly-die-qsl760jr9 [Accessed 6 April 2020].

Soldatkin, V. (2020) 'Moscow rolls out Sputnik V COVID-19 vaccine to most exposed groups', *Reuters*, 5 December, Available from: www.reut ers.com/article/health-coronavirus-russia-vaccination-idUSKBN28F09G [Accessed 15 December 2020].

Social Science Space (2020) 'Addressing the psychology of "Together Apart": free book download', blog, Available from: www.socialsciencesp ace.com/2020/05/addressing-the-psychology-of-together-apart-free-book-download/ [Accessed 15 December 2020].

Spiegelhalter, D.J., Aylin, P., Best, N.G. et al (2002) 'Commissioned analysis of surgical performance using routine data: lessons from the Bristol inquiry', *Journal of the Royal Statistical Society* A 165(2): 191–231, Available from: https://rss.onlinelibrary.wiley.com/doi/pdf/10.1111/1467-985X.02021 [Accessed 3 August 2021].

Spencer, B. and Lintern, S. (2022) 'This is what living with COVID looks like', *Sunday Times*, News section, 26 June, p. 12.

Spinney, L. (2018) *Pale Rider: The Spanish Flu of 1918 and how it changed the World*, London: Vintage.

Starkey, J. (2020) '1st Vets Railcard: Captain Sir Tom Moore award first veterans' railcard – to say thank you for his World War Two service', *The Sun*, 14 October, Available from: www.thesun.co.uk/news/12924131/capt ain-sir-tom-moore-awarded-first-veterans-railcard-to-say-thank-you-for-his-world-war-two-service/ [Accessed 15 December 2020].

Starr, P. (1982) *The Social Transformation of American Medicine: The Rise of a Sovereign Profession and the Making of a Vast Industry*, New York: Basic Books.

Sut, H.K. and Kucukkaya, B. (2020) 'Anxiety, depression, and related factors in pregnant women during the COVID-19 pandemic in Turkey: a web-based cross-sectional study', *Perspectives in Psychiatric Care*, 57(2): 860–8, Available from: https://onlinelibrary.wiley.com/doi/10.1111/ppc.12627 [Accessed 16 September 2021].

Swinford, S. (2020) 'Covid can be beaten but don't drop our guard, warns Jonathan Van-Tam', *The Times*, 10 November, Available from: https://www.thetimes.co.uk/article/coronavirus-can-be-beaten-but-don-t-drop-our-guard-warns-jonathan-van-tam-z8lj6l7nm [Accessed 16 August 2021].

Syed, M. (2020) 'Fixated on the flu and shrouded in secrecy, Britain's scientists picked the wrong remedy', *Sunday Times*, 17 May, p. 20.

Taiwan CDC (2018) 'NHCC', Available from: https://www.cdc.gov.tw/En/Category/MPage/gL7-bARtHyNdrDq882pJ9Q [Accessed 16 June 2022].

Tanay, M.A., Wiseman, T, Roberts, J. and Ream, E. (2013) 'A time to weep and a time to laugh: humour in the nurse–patient relationship in an adult cancer setting', *Supportive Care in Cancer*, 22: 1295–1301, Available from: https://link.springer.com/article/10.1007/s00520-013-2084-0 [Accessed 6 October 2021].

Tang, J.W., Li, Y., Eames, I. Chan, P.K.S. and Ridgway, G.L. (2006) 'Factors involved in the aerosol transmission of infection and control of ventilation in healthcare premises', *Journal of Hospital Infection*, 64(2): 100–14.

Taylor, A. (2020) 'As covid-19 cases surge, global study paints grim picture for elder-care homes', *Washington Post*, 16 October, Available from: www.washingtonpost.com/world/2020/10/15/long-term-elder-care-coronavirus-nursing-homes-research-lessons/ [Accessed 15 December 2020].

The Telegraph (2020) '50 years of drink driving campaigns', *The Telegraph*, Available from: www.telegraph.co.uk/motoring/ road-safety/11215676/50-years-of-drink-driving-campaigns.html [Accessed 30 July 2020].

Thorne, L. (2020) 'White House coronavirus advisor Anthony Fauci praises Victorian attitude to mask wearing', ABC News, 28 October, Available from: www.abc.net.au/news/2020-10-28/white-house-covid-expert-anthony-fauci-praises-victoria-masks/12823856 [Accessed 15 December 2020].

Topping, A. (2021) 'What the Cummings whiteboard reveals about the Covid response', *The Guardian*, 26 May, Available from: https://www.theguardian.com/world/2021/may/26/what-the-cummings-whiteboard-reveals-about-the-covid-response [Accessed 19 August 2021].

Trump, D. (2016) 'Wow! I hear you Warren, Michigan. Streaming live - join us America. It is time to DRAIN THE SWAMP!', *Twitter*, 31 October, Available from: https://twitter.com/realDonaldTrump/status/79319330219272198?ref_src=twsrc%5Etfw%7Ctwcamp%5Etweetembed%7Ctwterm%5E793193310219272198%7Ctwgr%5Eda1cd792f76941988fcd0ee77d7370032c4347da%7Ctwcon%5Es1_&ref_url=https%3A%2F%2Fmetro.co.uk%2F2018%2F01%2F20%2Fwhat-does-drain-the-swamp-mean-and-why-did-donald-trump-say-it-7245279%2F [Accessed 21 December 2022].

Trump, D. (2020) 'Remarks by President Trump in Press Briefing, April 14 2020', Available from: https://it.usembassy.gov/remarks-by-president-trump-in-press-briefing-april-14-2020/ [Accessed 2 February 2022].

UK Parliament (2021) *Coronavirus Pandemic (COVID-19): Inquiries and Reports*, Available from: https://www.parliament.uk/business/publications/coronavirus/inquiries-and-reports/ [Accessed 30 January 2022].

Ullah, H.K. (2017) *Digital World War: Islamists, Extremists and the Fight for Cyber Supremacy*, New Haven, CT and London: Yale University Press.

uPolitics (2020) 'Trump calls Dr. Anthony Fauci an "idiot," considers firing him', MSN News, 19 October, Available from: www.msn.com/en-us/news/politics/trump-calls-dr-anthony-fauci-an-idiot-considers-firing-him/ar-BB1abBHA [Accessed 15 December 2020].

Urwin, R. (2021) 'Baby, it was nearly too much to bear', *Sunday Times*, News Review, p. 24.

USA Today (2020) 'The full transcript from the first presidential debate between Joe Biden and Donald Trump', *USA Today*, 30 September, Available from: https://eu.usatoday.com/story/news/politics/elections/2020/09/30/presidential-debate-read-full-transcript-first-debate/3587462001/ [Accessed 15 December 2020].

van der Molen, M. and Brown, P. (2021) 'Following Dutch healthcare professionals' experiences during COVID-19: tensions in everyday practices and policies amid shifting uncertainties', *Current Sociology Monograph*, 69(4): 453–70.

Wahliquist, C. (2021) 'Australian ad showing Covid patient gasping for air "could increase vaccine hesitancy"', *The Guardian*, 12 July, Available from: https://www.theguardian.com/australia-news/2021/jul/12/australian-ad-showing-covid-patient-gasping-for-air-could-increase-vaccine-hesitancy [Accessed 2 December 2022].

Walach, H., Klement, R.J. and Aukema, W. (2021) 'The safety of COVID-19 vaccinations – we should rethink the policy', *Vaccines*, 9(7): 693, Available from: https://www.mdpi.com/2076-393X/9/7/693/htm [Accessed 5 September 2022].

Wan, W. (2020) 'America is running short on masks, gowns and gloves. Again', 9 July, *Washington Post*, Available from: https://www.washingtonpost.com/health/2020/07/08/ppe-shortage-masks-gloves-gowns/ [Accessed 18 March 2021].

Wang, C.J., Ng, C.Y. and Brook, R.H. (2020) 'Response to COVID-19 in Taiwan: big data analytics, new technology, and proactive testing', *JAMA*, 323(14): 1341–2.

Wang, D. and Mao, Z. (2021) 'From risks to catastrophes: how Chinese newspapers framed the coronavirus disease 2019 (COVID-19) in its early stage', *Health, Risk & Society*, 23(3–4): 93–110.

Ward, L. (2020) 'Covid 19 coronavirus: Auckland's dire August – the cluster that changed everything', *New Zealand Herald*, 7 September, Available from: www.nzherald.co.nz/nz/news/article.cfm?c_id=1&objec-tid=12362661 [Accessed 15 December 2020].

Ward, P.R., Foley, K., Meyer, S.B. Thomas, J., Huppatz, E., Olver, I. Miller, E.R. and Lunnay, B. (2022) 'Uncertainty, fear and control during COVID-19 ... or ... making a safe boat to survive rough seas: the lived experience of women in South Australia during early COVID-19 lockdowns', in P.R. Brown and J. Zinn (eds) *Covid-19 and the Sociology of Risk and Uncertainty: Studies of Social Phenomena and Social Theory Across 6 Continents*, Basingstoke: Springer Nature, pp 167–90.

Watson, G. (2019) 'The anti-vaccination movement that gripped Victorian England', 28 December, Available from: https://www.bbc.co.uk/news/uk-england-leicestershire-50713991 [Accessed 14 January 2022].

Weaver, M. (2020) 'Doctor who pleaded for more hospital PPE dies of coronavirus', *The Guardian*, 9 April, Available from: https://www.theguardian.com/world/2020/apr/09/consultant-who-pleaded-for-more-nhs-hospital-ppe-dies-of-coronavirus [Accessed 8 March 2021].

Wei, S. Q., Bilodeau-Betrand, M., Liu, S. and Auger, N. (2021) 'The impact of COVID-19 on pregnancy outcomes: a systematic review and meta-analysis', *CMAJ*, 193(16): E540–E548, Available from: https://www.cmaj.ca/content/193/16/E540 [Accessed 15 September 2021].

Whaley, F. (2006a) 'Solving the Metropole Hotel mystery', in WHO (ed.) *SARS: How a Global Epidemic was Stopped*, Geneva: WHO, pp 141–8, Available from: https://apps.who.int/iris/bitstream/handle/10665/207501/9290612134_eng.pdf [Accessed 4 November 2021].

Whaley, F. (2006b) 'Lockdown at Amoy Gardens', in WHO (ed.) *SARS: How a Global Epidemic was Stopped*, Geneva: WHO, pp 155–62, Available from: https://apps.who.int/iris/bitstream/handle/10665/207501/9290612134_eng.pdf [Accessed 4 November 2021].

The White House (2020a) 'Remarks by President Trump, Vice President Pence, and members of the Coronavirus Task Force in press conference', 26 February, Available from: https://trumpwhitehouse.archives.gov/briefings-statements/remarks-president-trump-vice-president-pence-members-coronavirus-task-force-press-conference/ [Accessed 14 December 2021].

The White House (2020b) 'Remarks by President Trump, Vice President Pence, and members of the Coronavirus Task Force in press briefing', 29 March, Available from: https://trumpwhitehouse.archives.gov/briefings-statements/remarks-president-trump-vice-president-pence-members-coronavirus-task-force-press-briefing-14/ [Accessed 16 February 2022].

The White House (2021) 'Statement by President Joe Biden on the investigation into the origins of COVID-19, statements and releases', 26 May, Available from: https://www.whitehouse.gov/briefing-room/statements-releases/2021/05/26/statement-by-president-joe-biden-on-the-investigation-into-the-origins-of-covid-19/ [10 July 2021].

Whyte, L. (2016) 'Sierra Leone: Ebola crisis sparks teen pregnancy surge as girls face sexual exploitation', *International Business Times*, updated 22 June, Available from: https://www.ibtimes.co.uk/sierra-leone-ebola-crisis-sparks-teen-pregnancy-surge-girls-face-sexual-exploitation-1566470 [Accessed 13 May 2020].

WHA (2020) '73rd World Health Assembly, Agenda Item 3, COVID-19 response', 19 May, Available from: https://apps.who.int/gb/ebwha/pdf_files/WHA73/A73_R1-en.pdf [Accessed 21 July 2021].

WHO (1978) 'Declaration of Alma-Ata, International Conference on Primary Health Care, Alma-Ata, USSR, 6–12 September 1978', Available from: https://cdn.who.int/media/docs/default-source/documents/alma ata-declaration-en.pdf?sfvrsn=7b3c2167_2 [Accessed 13 October 2021].

WHO (2020a) 'WHO Director-General's statement on IHR Emergency Committee on Novel Coronavirus (2019-nCoV)', WHO, 30 January, Available from: https://www.who.int/director-general/speeches/detail/who-director-general-s-statement-on-ihr-emergency-committee-on-novel-coronavirus-(2019-ncov [Accessed 29 November 2021].

WHO (2020b) 'How is COVID spread and how to protect yourself against it', 28 February, Available from: https://www.facebook.com/WHO/vid eos/how-is-covid-19-spread-and-how-do-you-protect-yourself-against-it/507223210199209/ [Accessed 29 November 2021].

WHO (2020c) 'Transmission of SARS-CoV-2: implications for infection prevention precautions', scientific brief, 9 July, Available from: https://www.who.int/news-room/commentaries/detail/transmission-of-sars-cov-2-implications-for-infection-prevention-precautions [Accessed 26 November 2020].

WHO (2020d) 'Shortage of personal protective equipment endangering health workers worldwide', 3 March, Available from: https://www.who.int/news/item/03-03-2020-shortage-of-personal-protective-equipment-endangering-health-workers-worldwide#:~:text=The%20World%20Hea lth%20Organization%20has%20warned%20that%20severe,from%20the%20new%20coronavirus%20and%20other%20infectious%20diseases [Accessed 18 March 2021].

WHO (2020e) 'Modes of transmission of virus causing COVID-19: implications for IPC precaution recommendations', scientific brief, 7 March, WHO, Available from: https://apps.who.int/iris/bitstream/han dle/10665/331601/WHO-2019-nCoV-Sci_Brief-Transmission_modes-2020.1-eng.pdf?sequence=1&isAllowed=y [Accessed 26 November 2021].

WHO (2020i) 'Mask use in the context of COVID-19, Interim Guidance', WHO, 1 December, Available from: https://www.who.int/publications/i/item/advice-on-the-use-of-masks-in-the-community-during-home-care-and-in-healthcare-settings-in-the-context-of-the-novel-coronavi rus-(2019-ncov)-outbreak [Accessed 29 November 2021].

WHO (2021a) 'Tracking SARS-CoV-2 variants', Available from: https://www.who.int/en/activities/tracking-SARS-CoV-2-variants/ [Accessed 14 July 2021].

WHO (2021b) 'WHO Academy', Available from: https://www.who.int/about/who-academy [Accessed 13 October 2021].

WHO (2021c) 'Roadmap to improve and ensure good indoor ventilation in the context of COVID-19', WHO, Available from: https://www.who.int/publications/i/item/9789240021280 [Accessed 29 November 2021].

WHO (2021d) 'COVID-19 Virtual Press conference transcript – 9 February 2021', Available from: https://www.who.int/publications/m/item/covid-19-virtual-press-conference-transcript---9-february-2021 [Accessed 2 February 2022].

WHO (2021e) 'WHO-convened global study of origins of SARS-CoV-2: China part, joint WHO–China study, 14 January–10 February 2021, joint report', WHO, 30 March, Available from: https://www.who.int/publications/i/item/who-convened-global-study-of-origins-of-sars-cov-2-china-part [Accessed 3 February 2022].

WHO (2022) 'Infodemic', Available from: https://www.who.int/health-topics/infodemic#tab=tab_1 [Accessed 20 August 2022].

Wikipedia (2020) 'QAnon', Available from: https://en.wikipedia.org/wiki/QAnon [Accessed 1 December 2020].

Wilson, S. (2020) 'Three reasons why Jacinda Ardern's coronavirus response has been a masterclass in crisis leadership', *The Conversation*, 5 April, Available from: https://theconversation.com/three-reasons-why-jacinda-arderns-coronavirus-response- has-been-a-masterclass-in-crisis-leadership-135541 [Accessed 15 December 2020].

Wong, J.C. (2020) 'Down the rabbit hole: how QAnon conspiracies thrive on Facebook', *The Guardian*, 25 June, Available from: https://www.theguardian.com/technology/2020/jun/25/qanon-facebook-conspiracy-theories-algorithm [Accessed 5 December 2022].

Wood, N. (2020) 'New Zealand's renewed COVID crisis: why scientists say the virus is hard to contain', 19 August, Available from: https://abcnews.go.com/Health/zealands-renewed-covid-crisis-scientists-virus-hard/story?id=72420563 [Accessed 15 December 2020].

Woodward, B. (2020a) *Rage*, London and New York: Simon & Schuster.

Woodward, A. (2020b) 'Coronavirus: scientists advised against hand-shakes on day Boris Johnson boasted of "shaking hands continuously"', 5 May, Available from: www.independent.co.uk/news/uk/politics/coronavirus-boris-johnson-hand-shake-scientists-a9499976.html [Accessed 15 December 2020].

Yang, T. U., Noh, J. Y., Song, J.-Y. et al (2021) How lessons learned from the 2015 Middle East respiratory syndrome outbreak affected the response to coronavirus disease 2019 in the Republic of Korea, The *Korean Journal of Internal Medicine*, 36(2): 271–85, Available from: https://www.kjim.org/journal/view.php?doi=10.3904/kjim.2020.371 [Accessed 17 June 2022].

YouTube (2020a) Boris Johnson on *This Morning*, 5 March, Available from: www.youtube.com/watch?v=vOHiaPwtGl4 [Accessed 18 August 2021].

YouTube (2020b) 'Coronavirus press conference (30 April 2020)', Available from: https://www.youtube.com/watch?v=T6qBIiBPjuA [Accessed 15 December 2020].

YouTube (2020c) '76 Days: inside Wuhan's lockdown', Available from: https://www.youtube.com/watch?v=_0LgdWg02D4? [Accessed 5 December 2022].

YouTube (2020d) 'Trump returns to the White House after COVID-19 treatment', Available from: www.youtube.com/watch?v=4eGrBei8HP4 [Accessed 5 December 2022].

Zadrozny, B. (2021) ' "Carol's Journey": what Facebook knew about how it radicalized users', NBC News, 22 October, Available from: https://www.nbcnews.com/tech/tech-news/facebook-knew-radicalized-users-rcna3581 [Accessed 13 January 2022].

Zahawi, N. (2021) 'Minister Nadhim Zahawi Oral Statement [to Parliament] on step 4 of the road map', 19 July, Available from: https://www.gov.uk/government/speeches/minister-nadhim-zahawi-oral-statement-on-step-4-of-the-road-map [Accessed 25 August 2021].

Zinn, J.O. (2008) 'Heading into the unknown: everyday strategies for managing risk and uncertainty', Health, Risk & Society, 10(5): 439–45.

Index

Note: References to tables appear in **bold** type.

5G, linked to the coronavirus outbreak in Wuhan 126–7
9/11 attacks 135, 136
76 Days: Inside Wuhan's Lockdown 100
737 Max 11
1918–1919 flu pandemic 15, 95–6

A

ABC News 109–10
Abdulwahab, Ismail Mohamed 108
Adams, Mark 112–13
Advisory Committee on Immunization Practices (ACIP)/US 42
aerosol spray, virus spread by 78–9, 80–1, 82, 84, 85, 157–8
Africa 14, 19, 68
Africa Centres for Disease Control and Prevention 68
African Union 68
Agyapong, Mary 114
Ahmed, Ibrahim Datti 121
AIDS/HIV pandemic 60
air travel 12
Alaszewski, A. 48, 60, 88
alert system
  New Zealand 55, **56–7**, 58
  UK 53
Alpha variant 25
American Psychiatric Association 7
Andrade, G. 120, 120–1
anti-vax movement 125–6, 129–30
anxiety 39, 41
Aptaclub 40
Ardern, Jacinda 55, 58, 59, 134, 156
al-Arefe, Mohammed 122
Armstrong, D. 7
Aronowitz, R.A. 7, 11
Ashworth, E. 40
Astra Zeneca vaccine 19
asylums 6
asymptomatic transmission 27
Audet, C. 40
Australia 13–14, 19–20, 39, 47, 134
authority, lack of unified 119
autistic people 142
Awan, Imran 122–3
Azur, Alex 70

B

Bahrain 18–19
Bal, J. 92–3
Bal, R. 92–3
BAME (Black and minority ethnic) communities 31, 113–15, 142
Barr et al 115
bats, most likely source of the virus 146, 148
Beck, Ulrich xii, 4, 5, 8, 119, 120
Belgium 40
Biden, Joe 114, 149
Birx, Deborah 71, 76
Black Africans, and vaccine hesitancy 61
Black Americans 114–15
Black Caribbeans, and vaccine hesitancy 61
Black Lives Matter 114
blame 5, 142, 144, 145, 150
  from inquiries 136, 138, 161
Boeing 11
Bolsonaro, Jair 119, 138
Bourdieu, P. 87
Bousso, Dr Abdoulaye 69
Bowbelle 135
Brazil 18, 119, 138, 157
Brearley, Joeli 112
Brexit 123
Bristol Royal Infirmary 12, 136
British Columbia 82–3
British Columbian Nursing Union (BCNU) 82
British Medical Association (BMA) 34
Brown, Ian 132–3
Brown, P. 3, 85, 94, 95
BSE (Bovine Spongiform Encephalopathy) 5, 67
bubonic plague 104–5, **105**
Burgess, A. 6, 120

C

California 32
Calnan, M. 3
Calvez, M. 60–1
Campbell, A. 136
Camus, Albert 105
Canada 26, **31**, 35–6, 82
Canadian Commission 136
Canadian Institute for Health Information 36

cancer 30, 92, 120
cardiovascular disease 12, 30, **35**, 90
care homes 35–6, 37, 44, 108,
    112–13, 142
Caserotti et al 62
Center for Disease Control and Prevention
    (CDC)/South Korea 13
CDC (Center for Disease Control and
    Prevention)/US 42, 59, 70, 78, 96–7
    guidance on mask wearing 71, 132
Central Epidemic Command Centre
    (Taiwan) 50
childbirth 88
children
    low risk of serious illness 32
    vaccination of 77
China 14–15, 16, 18, 157
    vaccination priorities 41, 43
    and zero-COVID policy 152
China National Health Commission 145
Chinese Coronavirus Epidemiology
    Team 29–30
Chowdhury, Abdul Mahud 99
Chung, Samantha 111
Clark, Helen 146
Clarke, Rachel 90, 92, 98–100, 105–6
Clarke et al 136
Coalition of Epidemic Preparedness
    Innovations (CEPI) 148
COBRA/COBR (Civil Contingencies
    Committee) 21–2, **73**, 75–6
Cochrane, Archie 83
Coderey, C. 86–7
cognitive dissonance 26–7
conspiracy theories 84, 120–31, 133–4,
    155, 160–1
contact tracing 14, 15
Conte, Giuseppe 134
Coronavirus Action Plan (UK) 21
Coronavirus Task Force (US) 97
COVID-19
    Decision Support Tool **35**
    droplet versus aerosol spray 78–84
    effect on ethnic groups 113–15, 160
    framing 12–17, 151–3, 161
    possible causes of the initial
        outbreak 145–6
    risk of 29–32
    vaccines 41–5
    see also deaths; hospitals; zero-COVID
        policies
Creasy, Stella 112
Cremona general hospital 17
Creutzfeldt–Jakob disease (CJD) 5, 67
Cummings, Dominic 2, 33, 53, 76,
    138–40
Cunningham, S. 62
Cygnus 16
Czech Republic 128

D
Daszuk, Peter 148–9
Davies, Sally 16
Day, Joan 113
deaths 18, 27, 29, 51, 142, 153
    in care homes 35–6, 112, 113
    deciding what level was tolerable 46
    ethnic groups 113–14
    excess 23, 30, 36, 90
Decision Support Tool for COVID-19 **35**
Deeny, S. 114
Defoe, Daniel 105, 115
Delta variant 24, 25
depression 39, 41
deviance, social 6
diabetes 30
*Diagnostic and Statistical Manual of Mental
    Disorders* (American Psychiatric
    Association) 7
Dibben, M.R. 89
disease
    monitoring 13
    and risk 7
doctors, and interaction with patients 89
Douglas, Mary xii, 4, 5, 8, 60–1,
    135, 161
droplets, virus spread by 78, 79, 80, 82,
    83, **83**, 85

E
Eat Out to Help Out 77
Ebola 12, 49–50, 62–3, 68, 148, 161
    and conspiracy theories 127
    effect on women 38–9
    in the US 96
Ebright, Richard 148–9
economic risks, lack of interaction with
    health risks 76
Ejaz et al 121
Elston et al 39
Elwell-Sutton, T. 114
Embarek, Peter 146
emotional appeals 3
England, attendance at emergency
    departments during the
    pandemic 90
Enlightenment 1, 4
Equatorial Guinea 19
Estonia 49
ethnic minorities
    and COVID-19 113–15, 142, 160
    and vaccine hesitancy 61
excess deaths 23, 30, 36, 90
experts
    attacked by populists 123–4, 137
    mistrust in 127–9
    and risk 67
    trusted more than politicians 53, 156

F

Faccin et al 129, 130
face masks *see* masks
Fage-Butler, A.M. 117
Farrar, Sir Jeremy 21, 27, 77
Fatima, M. 121
Fauci, Anthony 54, 60, 70, 71,
 123, 133
fear 4, 40, 94, 105, 126
 and conspiracy theorists 160
 of mobile phone masts 120
Ferguson, Professor Neil 77
Fifield, A. 90
Figueiredo, C.M.S. 118–19
first-order observers 48, 116
Floyd, George 114
flu 12, 15–17, 22, 27, 30
 COVID-19 framed as 21, 26, 63,
  152, 161
 pandemic, 1918–1919 15, 95–6
 and vaccination 44, 155
Foucault, Michel 4, 6, 7, 8
framing 11–17, 21, 26, 49–50, 62–3,
 151–3, 161
France 26, 42, 43, 61, 129–30, 138
Francis, Gavin 92, 105
Frank, D.A. 116
Freeman, Makia 126–7
front-line workers 31, 43, 110
 ethnic minorities 114, 142, 160
 without PPE 99, 108, 159

G

Gabe, M. 4
gambling 28
gay community 60–1
gender, as risk factor for COVID-19 30
Germany 42, 43–4
Ghebreyesus, Tedros 107
Giddens, Anthony 1, 8, 103,
 119, 156
 on serious illness 87–8
 and reflexivity 4
Global North, and conspiracy
 theories 120, 122–7
Global South, and conspiracy
 theories 120–2
Gluckman, Peter 149
Goffman, E. 11
Gove, Michael 123
Graaff de, B. 92–3
Great Barrington Declaration 32
Green, J. 135
Greenhalgh et al 81, 82–3
Griffiths, Mark 34
Griglio, E. 137
The Guardian 111–12, 115
Gulf states 18–19

H

Haddon, C. 75, 76, 78
Hahn, Stephen 71
Haider et al 18
Hallett, Baroness Heather 138
Halpern, David 21
Hancock, Matt 19, 21, 85, 108, 140
hand hygiene 52
Hanoi 79
Harden, Anthony 112
harm, minimising 45
Harries, Dr Jenny 72, 76
Harries, T. 26
Hassan, Samia Suluhu 69
health care, and risk 158–9
Health Foundation 114
Health Security Agency (UK) 72
heart disease 30, **35**, 90
 paediatric heart surgery 12, 136
Heneghan, Carl 53
herd immunity 19, 26, 27, 32–3, 141
 and Vallance 21–2
 and wait and see approach 16
Heyman et al **41**
high-income countries 18–19, 46, 69,
 70–8, 154
 and health care 158, 159
Hipkins, Chris 20
Hitoshi Oshitani 81
HIV/AIDS pandemic 60
Holt, Alison 112
Hong Kong 20–1, 79, 80, 152
Honigsbaum, M. 127
hope 3, 19, 94, 100, 158
Horii, M. 6
Horlick-Jones, T. 48, 89
Horton, Richard 21
hospitals
 discharge of patients to care homes
  without testing 36, 37
 during the pandemic 89–94, 95
 pressure on 17, 23, 25–6, 33–4, 36–7, 158
House of Commons Committee on Health
 and Social Care 127–8, 138–42
House of Commons Science and
 Technology Committee 76, 77–8,
 127–8, 138–42
Hungary 128
Hussain, A. 121
Hussain, S.A. 121
hypertension 30

I

Icke, David 126
illness, serious *see* serious illness
Independent Scientific Pandemic Insights
 Group on Behaviours (SPIB)/UK 52
Indonesia 43

infectious disease
  experts 83
  monitoring 13
influencers 118, 122
influenza *see* flu
Influenza Preparedness Programme
  (UK) 97, 98
infodemics 120
inquiries 135, 138–9, 161
  BRI Inquiry 12, 136
  BSE Inquiry 67
  Ischgl and Paznaun valley inquiry 142–4
  public 135–7, 138
  WHO inquiries 145–9, 150
Intelligence Community (IC)/US 149
intensive care facilities, triaging 34–5, 153
International Science Council (ISC) 149
intimate societies 86–7, 89
Ischgl and Paznaun valley inquiry 142–4
Islamophobia 122–4
isolation 40, 41
Italy 17, 34, 91, 134
Ittefaq, M. 121

J

Jabs (anti-vaccine campaign group) 125–6
Jamal, Tariq 122
Japan 5–6, 15, 18, 50–1, 63, 96
  on aerosol transmission 80–1, 84, 157
Jawed, Mohammed 110
JCVI (Joint Committee on Vaccination and
  Immunisation)/UK 46, **74**, 75, 77, 140
  on vaccination priorities 42, 44–5,
  154–5
Jenner, Edward 125
Jennings et al 134
Jetten et al 47–8
Johns Hopkins University 18
Johnson, Boris 23, 25, 51–2, 53, 132, 134
  claimed to be 'following the science' 72
  and COBRA 76
  favoured letting the virus spread 21
  lifted all legal limits on social contacts in
    England 24
  on Omicron 109
Jurich, E.K. 117–18

K

Kaiser, C. 124
Kewell, B.J. 12
key workers 43
Khan-Williams, Roxana 122–3
Kierney, Dorothy 113
Kiisel, M. 48–9
Kilbourne, E.D. 16
Kondor, K. 128, 129
Korea, South 13, 18
Kriesi, H. 123
Kucukkaya, B. 39

L

Lacey, Richard 5
large-scale societies 89
Larrey, Dominique Jean 28–9
Lean, M. 89
learning disabilities, people with 142
Learn the Risk 126
Lebela et al 39–40
legislative committees 137–8
Lewis, G. 86
Liberia 68
Lima, Peru 17
Li Wenliang 94, 103
lockdown 2, 37, 105, 153, 160
  definition 18
  breach of rules 11, 53, 58, 59, 63, 76, 77
  Australia 39
  New Zealand 20, 55, 58
  UK 22–4, 27, 52, 53, 141
  US 54, 71
  Wuhan 14–15, 16, 18, 34
Lombardy, Italy 91
low-income countries 19, 68
Luhmann, N. 48
Lupton, D. 5

M

Magaufuli, President John 69
Mairal, G. 105
Makoto Tsubokura 80–1
Malta 18
Mao, Z. 14
Marchioness 135–6
Maria Auxiliadora hospital, Lima 17
masks 50, 54, 69, 71, 79, 109
  to help prevent aerosol transmission 85,
    157, 158
  in Japan 5–6, 51, 81, 96
  resistance to 132–3
  and WHO guidance 84, 131–2
Masood, Mufti 122
mass media, compared with social
  media 118–19
Matar et al 37
maternal deaths 39
Mchembe, Dr 69
measles, mumps and rubella (MMR)
  vaccine 125
media
  mass compared with social media 118–19
  on COVID-19 110–13
  on risk 103–4
medical and health research funding 69,
  70, 72
Melo, T. de 118–19
mental disorder 6, 7
MERS (Middle East Respiratory
  Syndrome) 12, 13

Michigan 124
middle-income countries 68, 69
midwives 88
Mi Feng 145
Mihelj, S. 128, 129
Millennium Bug 47
mistrust 53, 62, 119, 127–8
mobile phone masts 120
modernity 1, 103
Mogelson, L. 124
Mohdin, A. 111
Molen, M. van der 85, 94, 95
Montgomery, Sir Jonathan 34
Moore, Captain Tom 108, 110–11, 116, 160
Moral and Ethical Advisory Group (UK) 34
Morgan, Piers 60
Morrison, Scott 134
mortuaries 17
mothers 117–18
Mulkay, M.J. 84
Murphy, Brendan 14
Muslims, blamed for the spread of COVID-19 122–3
Myanmar 86–7

N

Nanshan Zhong 14
Napoleonic Wars 28
National Institute for Health and Care Research (NIHR)/UK 72
National Institute for Health Care and Excellence (NICE)/UK 35
National Institute of Allergy and Virology (NIAV)/US 70, 78
National Institutes for Health (NIH)/US 70
National Public Health Institute Liberia (NPHIL) 68
neo-colonialism 120
NERVTAG **74**, 75
Netherlands 26, 61, 85, 92–4
New York 17, 91–2
New York Times (2021) vaccination tracker 18
New Zealand 18, 20, 55–9, 63, 152
NHS (National Health Service)
collapse of to be avoided 22
protecting at the expense of social care 113
Nice, A. 75, 76, 78
Nigeria 67–8, 121
Nigeria Centre for Disease Control and Prevention 67–8
Northwick Park Hospital, London 17, 34, 91
nurses, and interaction with patients 88

O

Obama, Barack 26–7
Obama, Michelle 115
older people
denied intensive care due to triaging 34–5, 153
infected in care homes 35–7, 112–13, 142
and vaccination 43, 154, 155
Olympics, 2020 15
Omicron 25, 109, 152, 153
Operation Gridlock 124
Organisation for Economic Co-operation and Development (OECD), on vaccination 61
outcomes
measuring and valuing 2
measuring the probability of 1–2
Oxford/Astra Zeneca vaccine 19

P

paediatric heart surgery 12, 136
Pakistan 120–1, 122
pandemics, flu 15–16, 95–6
Panorama, documentary on deaths in care homes 112–13
Papua New Guinea 86
partogram 88
Partygate 25
patients, and interaction with health-care professionals 88–9
Paton, Alexis 45
Pence, Mike 70
Peru 17
Philo et al 104
Pinel, Phillipe 6–7
plague, bubonic 104–5, 105
polio vaccine 120–1
politicians, trusted less than experts 53, 156
POLITIFACT 97
Pollack, Dr Marjorie 103–4
pollution 5–6
populism 120, 122–3
populist leaders 85, 134
PPE 95–100, 108, 159
precautionary principle 37, **41**, 120, 147, 154
pre-diabetes 7
pregnant women 39–41, 44, 111–12, 114
high risk of COVID-19 32, 37–8, 154
and use of social media 117
Presenti, Antonio 34
presymptomatic transmission 27
probability 1–2, 28, 45–6, 50, 88, 153, 161
of serious illness 30, 37
and stockpiling PPE 97
Procopius 104–5

ProMed 103–4
Public Accounts Committee (UK) 36
public health campaigns 47, 84
public health messaging 49–63, 70
public inquiries 135–7, 138
Putin, Vladimir 41

Q

QAnon 124
Qatar 19
Quigley, K.F. 47

R

randomised control trials (RCTs) 82–3
rational decision making 1, 2, 158
rationality 1, 2
Redfield, Robert 70, 71
reflexivity 4
Reicher, S.D. 48
residential homes 35–6, 44, 108, 112–13, 142
respiratory disease, chronic 30
Rev 52–3, 97
Reynard, David 120
right-wing populism 122–3
risk
  calculation of the probability of one or
    more outcomes 28, 153
  categorisation 30–7, 154
  of COVID-19 29–32
  and expert knowledge 67, 156–8
  health care, managing 158–9
  and the media 103–4
  multiple competing narratives of 159–60
  and PPE 100
  as probabilities expressed by
    numbers 116
  as a social construct 6
  and triaging 153–4
  and vaccination 154–5
  and work of health professionals 89
risk assessment 1–2, 3
risk communication 155–6
risk evaluation 1, 2, 4–8
risk messages, communication of 47–59
Risk Society 4, 8
risk work 89
R$_o$, use of 159
road map 24
Robinson, Tommy 123
Rohrer, Dr Ronald 143–4
Roth, J.A. 88, 96
Russian Federation 41, 42–3

S

SAGE (Scientific Advisory Group for
  Emergencies) 23, 72, **73**, 75, 76, 77
Salminen, Mika 33
Sanchez, Lizzy Torres 110
San Francisco 120

SARS (Severe Acute Respiratory
  Syndrome) 26, 27, 79–80
  framing COVID-19 as 12, 13, 49–50,
    62–3, 151–2, 161
  outbreak in Ontario 136
Sasse, T. 75, 76, 78
Saudi Arabia 122
Scamell, M. 88
Scientific American 54
scientific knowledge 84–5, 87, 89
scientific research 69, 70, 72
scientists
  in high-income countries 69, 70–8
  in low- and middle-income
    countries 68, 69
  and policy makers 69–78, 157
  role 67
second-order observers 48, 116
second wave 23, 24, 36, 77
Sedwill, Lord 137
self-isolating 30, **31**, **57**
Senegal 14, 69, 152, 157
Serbia 128
serious illness 30, 37, 86–9, 95, 158
  children and young adults lower risk 32
  risk of for front-line workers 159
Shane, T. 118
Shapps, Grant 110
shielding 30, **31**, 32
Shinzo Abe 15, 51, 156
Shi Zhengli 148
Sierra Leone 39
sin 5, 135
Singapore 79
Sirleaf, Ellen Johnson 146
Slovic, P. 116
smallpox vaccination 125
small-scale intimate societies 86–7, 89
'smouldering transmission' 152
social care 108, 113
social deviance 6
social distancing 14, 30, 50, 59
  in Japan 51
  in the UK 23, 24, 53, 132
social isolation 40, 41
social justice 44
social media 117–19, 124, 129–30
  and conspiracy theories 121–2, 133
  and vaccination 60
social relations, and vaccine hesitancy 62
South Korea 13, 18
Spanish flu 15, 95–6
SPI-B **74**
SPI-M **73**
Spinney, Laura 95–6
Stafford, M. 114
Starr, P. 7
Štětka, V. 128, 129
Stevens, Sir Simon 97–8

strangers, societies of 87
sub-Saharan Africa 19
Sunday Times 36
superspreading events 15, 20, 26, 27, 79, 81
Sut, H.K. 39
Sweden 32–3

T

Taiwan 13, 18, 50, 63, 152, 157
Tanay et al 88
Tanzania 69, 157
Taylor, A. 35
Tegnell, Anders 32–3
Tennant, Dr Rachel 91
Tesha, Wilbald 111
test and trace system 16, 141–2
testing, COVID-19 14, 108
Thalidomide 131
Toronto 79
transmission, smouldering 152
transparency 77, 85
triaging 28–9, 34–5, 153–4
Trump, President Donald 16–17, 54, 71, 78, 97, 107–8
  contested expert risk assessment and public health advice 123–4, 134, 137
  on mask wearing 133
  on WHO 123, 145
  and public health messaging 70
  and social media 118, 119
trust xiv, 2–3, 58, 63, 117, 134
  in experts 53, 127–9
  in messaging 48, 49
  patients' for doctors 89
  and risk communication 156
  undermined by behind closed doors decision making 155
  wearing PPE made it difficult to communicate with patients 159
trustworthiness 52, 62
Turkey 39
Twitter 119, 122, 129

U

UAE 18
UK
  on aerosol transmission 84
  and care home residents 36
  and conspiracy theories 127–8
  and COVID-19 in the media 110–13
  deaths 18
  guidance on mask wearing 132
  herd immunity strategy 33
  hospitals 34, 90, 91, 92
  households 87
  impact of COVID-19 on ethnic groups 114, 115
  inquiries into the pandemic 138–42

medical and health research funding 72
  planning for a pandemic focused on influenza 16
  policy 21–6, 27
  and PPE 97–9
  and pregnant women 40
  public health campaigns 47
  and public health messaging 51–3, 63
  regular televised briefings 108–9
  and risk categorisation **31**
  scientific community's links with policy makers poor 157
  scientific expertise 72–8
  and trust in government 134
  vaccination priorities 42, 44–5, 46
  and vaccine hesitancy 61
Ullah, H.K. 121
uncertainty, managing 3, 161
Urwin, Rosamund 40
US
  attendance at emergency departments during the pandemic 90
  citizens trusted health experts more than politicians 53
  and conspiracy theories 127
  excess death rate 30
  and 'flu frame' 16–17
  hospitals 91–2
  impact of COVID-19 on ethnic groups 113–15
  Johns Hopkins University 18
  and mask wearing 132, 133
  media narratives 109–10
  medical and health research funding 69, 70
  and the Millennium Bug 47
  and mobile phone masts 120
  and PPE 96–7
  and pregnant women 37–8
  and public health messaging 54, 63
  and risk categorisation 30–1
  scientific community's links with policy makers poor 157
  scientific expertise 70–1, 78
  and trust in government 134
  vaccination declined by one-third of military 60
  vaccination priorities 42
USNS *Comfort* 92

V

vaccination 18–19, 24, 25, 125–7, 140, 153
  booster jabs 109
  and conspiracy theories 124, 129–30, 160
  declined by one-third of US military 60
  in Hong Kong 20–1
  priorities 46, 154–5

vaccine hesitancy 61–2
vaccines 41–5, 59, 120–1
Vallance, Sir Patrick 21–2, 52–3, 75, 76, 140
value judgements 155
value system, triaging 153
Van-Tam, Jonathan 19, 72, 75, 76
Vastfjall, D. 116
ventilation, use of to reduce spread of
    COVID-19 79, 80, 84, 85, 157, 158
Vietnam 18
Vihalemm, T. 48–9
vulnerable individuals 43, 152–3, 161
  and vaccination 44, 45, 154, 155

W

wait and see policy 18, 27, 29, 52,
    152, 161
  and herd immunity policy 16, 33
  prioritised younger healthier people over
    older and vulnerable people 36
  threatened to overwhelm hospitals 158
Wakefield, Andrew 125, 126
Wan, W. 98
Wang, D. 14
Ward et al 39
Washington Post 98, 112
Wassan, Choudhary Aslam 115
Wassan, Zia 115
Wei et al 38
Wenliang, Dr Li 14
West Africa 14

White House Coronavirus Task Force 70
'White Male Effect' 62
Whitty, Chris 46, 52, 53, 72, 75, 132
  on intensive care 34
  on pregnant women 37
  on public inquiry 138
WHO (World Health Organization) 5, 14,
    16, 80, 81–2, 123
  guidance on mask wearing 83–4, 131–2
  on PPE 96, 98
  promotes global health 68
  two inquiries into COVID-19 145–50
Willis, Samantha 111–12
Winter Willow 16
women, pregnant *see* pregnant women
Woodward, A. 17
Woodward, B. 54, 70
Wuhan 13, 90–1, 103–4, 126
  lockdown 14–15, 16, 18, 34
Wyckoff Heights Medical Center,
    Brooklyn 17, 91–2

Y

YouTube 129

Z

Zahawi, Nadhim 24, 112
zero-COVID policies 27, 29, 58, 161
  in Australia 13–14, 19–20
  challenges 152
  in Japan 15